How does it feel?

The contributors

Ian Baker · Arthur Balaskas · Meirion Bowen · Wendy Campbell ·
Edmund Carpenter · Mick Csáky · Tom Falkner · Mick Gold · Richard L. Gregory ·
Bernard Gunther · David Hockney · Sharon Kretzmer · Ronald D. Laing ·
Edmund Leach · Edward Lucie-Smith · Philip Rawson · Charles Rycroft · Bani Shorter ·
David Tansley · Michael Tippett · Caroline Tisdall · Lyall Watson

with 227 illustrations
26 in color

Edited by Mick Csáky

How does it feel?

Exploring the world of your senses

H·A·R·M·O·N·Y B·O·O·K·S

New York

to Leo

Harmony Books, a division of Crown Publishers, Inc.
One Park Avenue, New York, N.Y. 10016

Library of Congress Cataloging in Publication Data
Main entry under title:

How does it feel?

   1. Senses and sensation.   2. Consciousness.
I. Csáky, Mick.
BF233.H64   1979   152.4   79-4510
ISBN 0-517-53829-6

Printed in Great Britain by BAS Printers Limited, Over Wallop, Hampshire
Color printed in Great Britain by Balding and Mansell Ltd, Wisbech
Filmset by Keyspools Ltd, Golborne, Lancs

Foreword

He who tastes not, knows not.
Jalaluddin Rumi

This book is about ways to explore and to celebrate the potential of our senses and emotions – our feelings. The theme of creative personal exploration, of heightened awareness and deeper feeling, runs through all twenty-three chapters. Leading authorities have been brought together to interpret these themes through their individual disciplines of psychology, physiology, anthropology, art, human growth techniques – and from basic common sense.

The question that has been in my mind during the preparation of this book has been: how does it feel to experience the world more directly and vividly – more authentically? My constant reference point has been a desire to achieve a more varied and intense awareness of the world in which I live, a desire that is hardly unique: to come to my senses.

There are five main sections in the book. The first, *Physiological Facts*, provides a physiological explanation of how we perceive the world, of how our sense organs function and how we make meaning of the world. In *Psychological Variety*, another approach is used to explain how and why our own personal idiosyncrasies colour the way in which we experience the world, so that we all experience it differently. *Social Conditioning* explores some of the many ways that people's senses and emotions are affected by the prevailing value systems within a culture, in a historical and anthropological context. The fourth section, *Sensory Enrichment*, is concerned with specific and practical ways in which we can heighten and enrich our feelings, through a greater appreciation of, and participation in, the arts. The last nine chapters, *Personal Potential*, are first-hand accounts from people who have achieved greater awareness and deeper feelings through some of the disciplines of the Human Growth movement, such as encounter, yoga, massage and bio-energetics; and finally through the recognition of a much wider frequency range of sensibilities embracing both mysticism and extrasensory perception.

Neither this book nor my film *How Does it Feel?* would have been made without the generous help of three people. It was Adrian Munsey who mapped out the basic structure from our early researches in America and Europe. His inventive imagination and knowledge of psychology and the arts provided an invaluable creative contribution. Rodney Wilson, of the Arts Council's Film Department, has given much support and encouragement. It was his initial interest in what was no more than a barely formed notion that led to my film, and consequently to this book. David Beatty is greatly responsible for the selection of visual and verbal illustrations that run through the book. I have relied upon his choice of poetry, prose, photography and paintings to help throw the ideas within each section and chapter into the broadest of contexts.

Mick Csáky

Contents

Foreword   5
'Feeling'   *Ronald D. Laing*   11
Experience is everything   *Mick Csáky*   17

PHYSIOLOGICAL FACTS:
how your senses work

Feeling the world by perception   *Richard L. Gregory*   55

PSYCHOLOGICAL VARIETY:
interpreting the world through your senses

The psyche and the senses   *Charles Rycroft*   69
Character and creativity   *Ian F. Baker*   77

SOCIAL CONDITIONING:
understanding cultural values

Of ecstasy and rationality   *Edmund Leach*   91
They became what they beheld   *Edmund Carpenter*   109
Taste and smell   *Edmund Leach*   119
Sensibility and history   *Edward Lucie-Smith*   125

SENSORY ENRICHMENT:
artists lead the way

Every human being is an artist   *Caroline Tisdall*   139
Painting a picture   *David Hockney*   149
Rock music and the senses   *Mick Gold*   153
Music of the mind and body   *Meirion Bowen*   163
Feelings of inner experience   *Michael Tippett*   173

PERSONAL POTENTIAL:
transforming your experience

Light out of darkness   *Bani Shorter*   183
Encounter   *Tom Falkner*   195
Primal therapy   *Wendy Campbell*   203
Massage   *Sharon Kretzmer*   211
Sensory awakening: Couples   *Bernard Gunther*   217
Body awareness   *Arthur Balaskas*   223
The senses of India and China   *Philip Rawson*   231
Extrasensory perception and healing   *David Tansley*   247
Many realities   *Lyall Watson*   257

Acknowledgements   263

IS THERE A LIFE

Their idols are silver and gold
The work of men's hands.
They have mouths, but they speak not;
Eyes they have, but they see not;
They have ears, but they hear not;
They have hands, but they handle not;
Feet they have, but they walk not;
Neither speak they through their throat.
Psalm 113

Either we want to live or we want to die, and while
we are alive we surely want to live more abun-
dantly, to fulfil our potential, to realise our capacities, instead of living a death in life. We can't be
fully alive if our feelings are dead. Our senses and
our feelings are our very experience of our aliveness. And as sentient living creatures it seems a
shame to miss the experience of life. And as living
creatures it seems only common sense to be
aware of ourselves and that means knowing how
we feel and what we feel and why we feel.
R. D. Laing

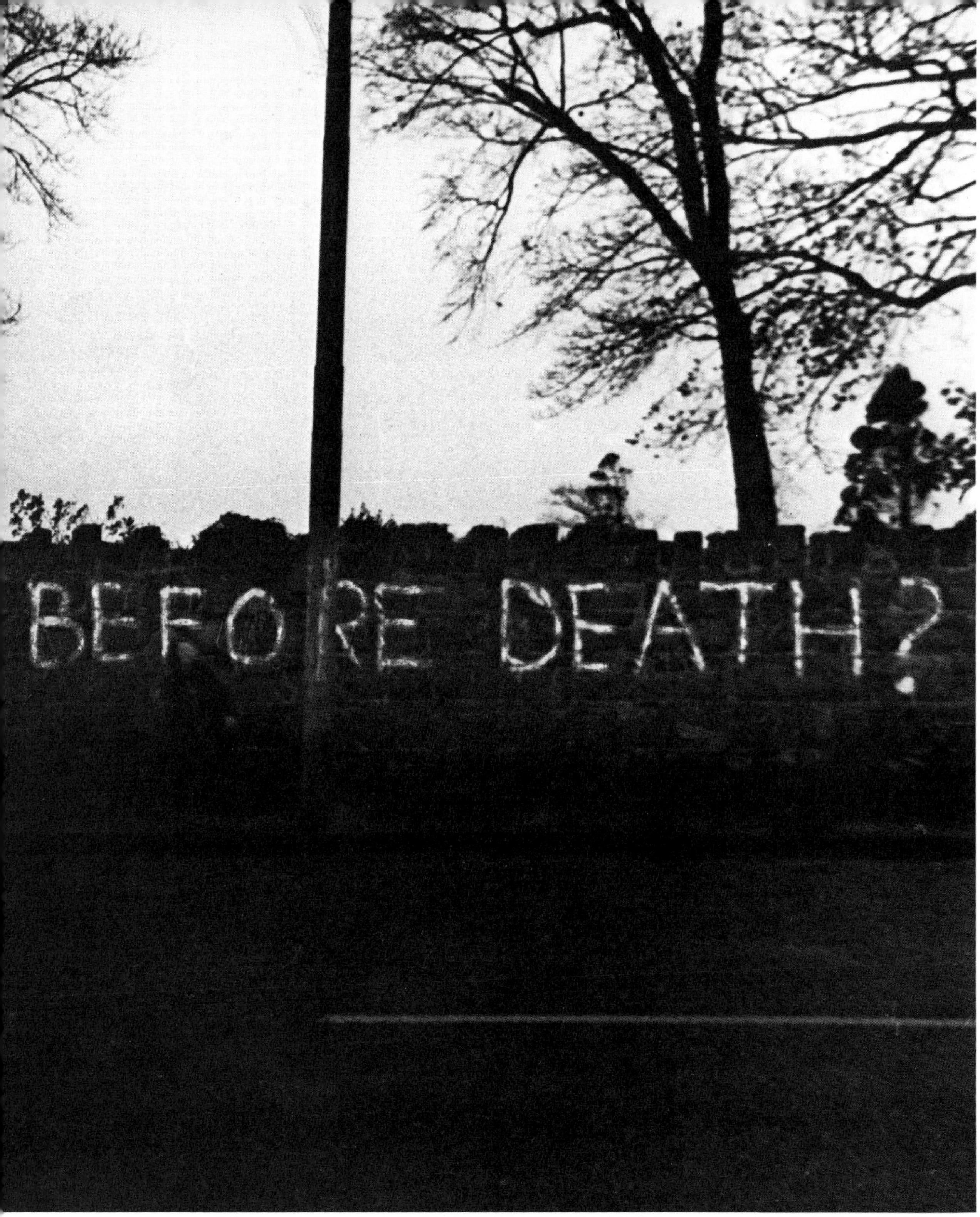
BEFORE DEATH?

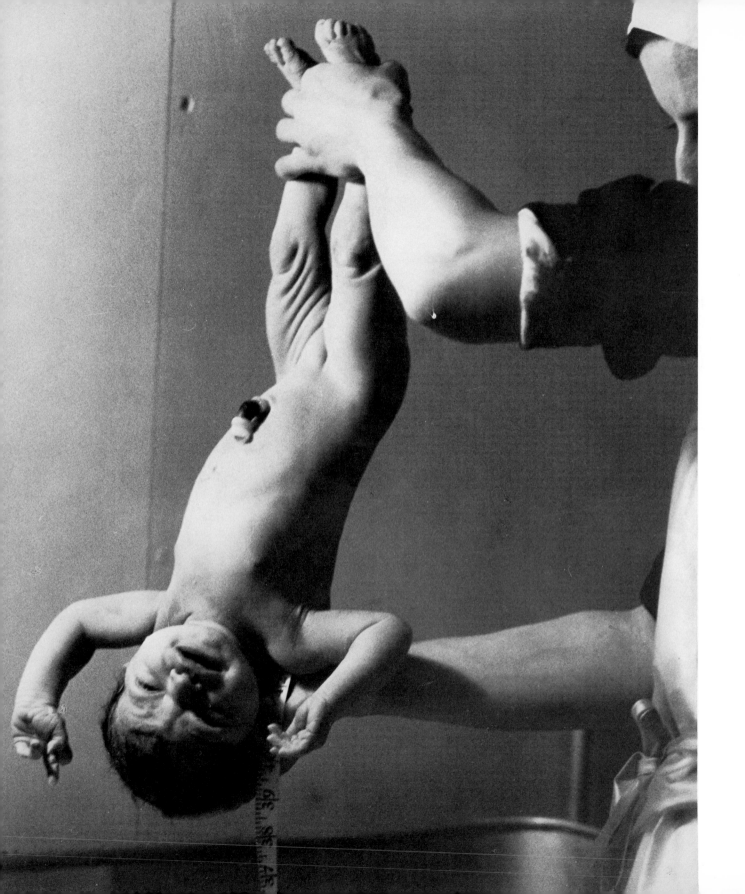

R. D. LAING

R. D. Laing is a psychiatrist and psychoanalyst, and author of several books including *The Divided Self*, *The Politics of Experience*, *Self and Others*, *The Facts of Life*, and *Do You Love Me?* He has conducted extensive research into the possibilities of inter-personal communication, drug-induced awareness, the disciplines of yoga and meditation, sensory deprivation, and currently into the possibility of pre-natal consciousness.

'Feeling'

I

We are sentient, feeling creatures. Anything perceived, imagined, thought, remembered is, ordinarily, felt.

Millions of people are dissatisfied with how they feel. They either feel that they don't feel enough, or that they feel too much, or that they don't like what they feel, or they are simply bored with their same old, tired, faded feelings and want to change them, like a suit of clothes, a car, a spouse, for other newer, fresher, more interesting feelings.

Millions of people buy millions of pills each year to stop feeling what they feel: to feel less, and often, ideally, nothing.

Millions of people engage in special practices in the hope of feeling *something*, or to feel more, or to feel differently.

II

A young man and young woman, students at an American university, ask me, 'Should we try to get in touch with our feelings now, or should we wait [two years] until we graduate?'

As a psychiatrist and psychoanalyst, I am consulted by people of all ages, women and men, of many nationalities, rich and poor, young and old, married or single, divorced or bereaved, from all religions, believers or not, over states of misery they are in, in relation to how they feel or do not feel.

The nuances of complaints against feeling are legion. I feel miserable. I feel depressed. I feel suicidal. I feel dead. I don't feel human. I feel frantic. I feel frightened. I feel bad. I feel spiteful, envious, jealous, angry, resentful. I feel too much or too little. I am persecuted by my feelings. I am out of contact with my feelings. I hate my feelings. I do not know what I feel. I feel the wrong things.

III

This book addresses itself to the question of how we feel, whether the feeling be of sensation, of emotion, or of the world as we experience it.

Sensations, emotions and our experiential world are all problem areas in the existence of us modern men, women and children.

There are internal and external, interpersonal and social ambiguities, paradoxes, conflicts, confusion, pain and misery over the state of how we sense, feel and experience the world.

Two sets of people are going to read this book: those who feel, and do not feel anything intrinsically wrong with how they feel as such, however unpleasant or painful some feelings may sometimes be. And, on the other hand, those who are at odds with their feelings. Of this group there are those who do not want to feel as they do, and want to change their feelings; those who feel nothing or next to nothing and want simply to feel, almost anything; and those who want to have as little contact with their feelings as possible. Ideally they would prefer to have nothing more to do with feeling; for them nothing is better than anything.

IV

Much cant surrounds feeling.

> *The feelings I don't have, I don't have.*
> *The feelings you don't have, you don't have.*
> *The feelings you say you have, you don't have.*
> *The feelings you would like us all to have, we*
>   *neither of us have.*
> *The feelings people ought to have, they never*
>   *have.*
> *If people say they've got feelings, you may be*
>   *pretty sure they haven't got them.*
> *So if you want either of us to feel anything at all you'd better abandon all idea of*
> *feelings altogether.*

D. H. Lawrence

Many of the feelings many people feel are *insufferable* to them. The *conflict* between what one ought to feel or what one ought not to feel and what one does or does not feel is insufferable. If one's feelings do not change, they have to be eliminated from – how one feels.

Then one comes to be preoccupied by feelings one denies, disavows, disassociates oneself from, feelings one rejects, repudiates. Feelings one wishes to eliminate, annihilate, deaden, expunge. Feelings one resents having to feel. Feelings one runs away from, tries to avoid, cringes from. Feelings one cannot stomach, feelings that nauseate one, feelings one can't swallow, that cannot sink in, feelings of horror and horrifying feelings, feelings that make one shudder, totter, stagger, quiver, that send pangs through one's marrow: intolerable feelings, unbearable feelings, *insufferable* feelings.

One lady said to me, 'When I make contact with my feelings (not everyday) they are nothing but jangled chords.'

An ordered formal interlace has become a tangled labyrinth. A proper formal order has become cacophonous, raucous, out of tune, out of key.

The self-tormented sinner who is the would-be saint. The bitterness of irreversible defeat, disgrace, dishonour, discredit in others' or one's own eyes. It is not for nothing that so many people take so many pills, and are prescribed so many, in order to stop feeling the feelings they have. They are in torment, their own self-torture. It is extraordinary that a person may be full of implacable hatred for himself, and yet have to come to *realize* this for a first time. And only then, possibly, forbear to continue with his own self-torture. Some people, however, are aware, only too aware, of hating themselves, and may mutilate or kill themselves out of sheer *felt* hatred.

V

Why are feelings so unacceptable to so many?

They are out of control, wild, painful, in conflict, forbidden, nasty, ugly. There is no acceptable way to express them.

Many feelings are acceptable but *some* feelings spoil the others. One feeling may *poison* the others. One feeling may be jealous or envious of another feeling. Thinking, imagination, intuition, may be at odds with one's feelings or coexist in friendly concord.

One's feeling life may not be integrated into the rest of one's life.

What one *feels* may be at odds with what one thinks, imagines, dreams, or believes, wishes, desires, hopes, cherishes.

Feelings may be spurned not only because they are agonizing, unpredictable, out of control, but also because to the logic of the head, they may seem to be a mere *senseless* nuisance. Why a *pang* for instance? What is its message, what does it connote?

One may feel suffocated in ordinary air.

I believe it to be an innocent pleasure hence I *feel* resentment that I was made to feel guilty and ashamed of it. I despise myself because I feel frightened when I *feel* pleasure. Hence I *feel* hopeless. I *feel* so disappointed in myself. I *feel* my life is not my own. I *feel* a coward, I *feel* helpless, I feel defeated, I *feel* demoralized, I *feel* I can't go on, I feel like killing myself, if I didn't *feel* dead already.

And beyond all that, there are even deeper reasons for choosing to keep away from feeling contact with the world. A young woman expressed the matter with unsurpassable succinctness and clarity, 'I put up static between me and my senses – all the time. If I didn't, *I would have to be here.*'

VI

Millions of people are tormented by an obscene void where feelings *should* be but are not. No way to *force* a feeling to *obey* one's desire, and present itself to us. Many people can conjure up feelings and even convince themselves that the feelings they *imagine* they have, are actual feelings they do have.

One has to decide whether to accept or reject how one feels. Whether to allow, to admit, to suffer one's feelings, be they of joy or sorrow, pleasure or pain, of callousness or of concern, or whether to disavow and repress them.

Many people, it seems to me, confuse how they feel with how they act. They do not clearly discriminate the two domains. It is one thing to allow oneself to feel like killing someone, and quite another matter to do so. Everyone's heart, I suspect, is capable, potentially, of feeling the highest and lowest, the utmost generosity and the narrowest meanness. No wise man, who knows his heart, will ever be self-righteous.

'How hollow heart and full of filth thou art,' exclaims Samuel Beckett. But we should be charitable to our own wretchedness, as well as to that of others.

It is clear that *everything* hinges on our *attitude* to our feelings. Is our attitude to our feelings in itself an open-hearted attitude? *Have we compassion for our passion?*

VII

To feel is desirable. To feel free to feel is desirable. It is good not to be afraid of one's feelings.

It is good to achieve control of one's conduct such that one need no longer be afraid of committing murder because one feels fury or rage. It is instructive to look at one's feelings of desire and aversion, to become aware of them and to become aware of one's judgments about them – shame, pride, guilt, self-righteousness.

It is useful to look at the moral/ethical/spiritual issues over feeling and conduct, and to arrive at a clear view of what line to take.

It is preferable to resolve to face conflicts between opposite feelings *consciously* – as everything else *consciously*.

To study the body without knowing how a sentient body like ours feels through knowing the feelings of one's own sentient physical self, is like a deaf man studying music from an oscillograph.

We need to feel to be able to make critical judgments. To believe that we can fully *know*, without feeling, is what one might call the *apathetic fallacy*. This is to believe that feeling, whether that of the knower or the known, *should* be left out. With feeling go values. Once these have been consigned to the irrelevant dirty bath water of subjectivism or projective subjectivism (the pathetic fallacy) how much is left of the baby of the reality, and indeed the reality of the baby?

At the same time, feelings cannot be their own final critical authority of their own validity, probity and social fitness.

Our intellect must *see* our passions and have its own freedom to think what it has to think about how we feel, just as our feelings should have the right to be *felt*. What one makes of what one feels is what makes the difference between saint and sinner, sage and fool. But the feeling must be there. I can't imagine a man or woman of any sagacity who does not *feel* his or her own heart throb in tune and in time with the throb of the heart of the universe.

I have alluded to the infinite variety of felt experience, and said little of the delight

14

the felt experience of this wonderful world can bring. This book redresses the balance. It does not shirk the torture many people live through, even without the blights of poverty, starvation, disease, cruelty. But it does not neglect to celebrate the joy and wonder of dance and song and symphony. The ego can be a home we can leave and return to, as well as a dungeon in a rotting prison. Our soul has wings, we can romp with dolphins. We live in the womb and at the same time in infinite space.

We're a long time dead. Life is for living. In these pages Mick Csaky has given us the taste and ever fresh tingle of how it can feel to be joyously alive.

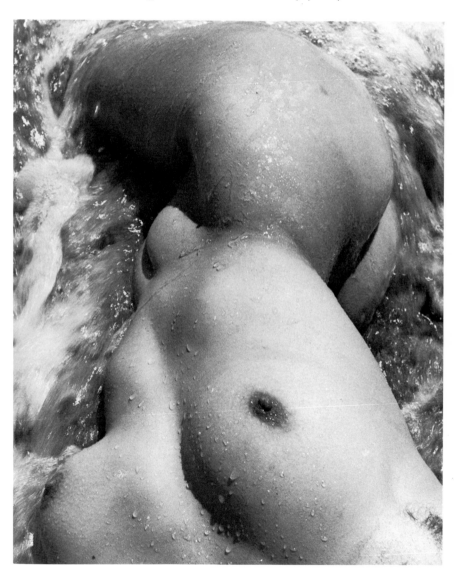

The great object of life is sensation – to feel that we exist, even though in pain. It is this 'craving void' which drives us to gaming – to battle – to travel – to intemperate, but keenly felt, pursuits of any description, whose principal attraction is the agitation inseparable from their accomplishment.
Byron

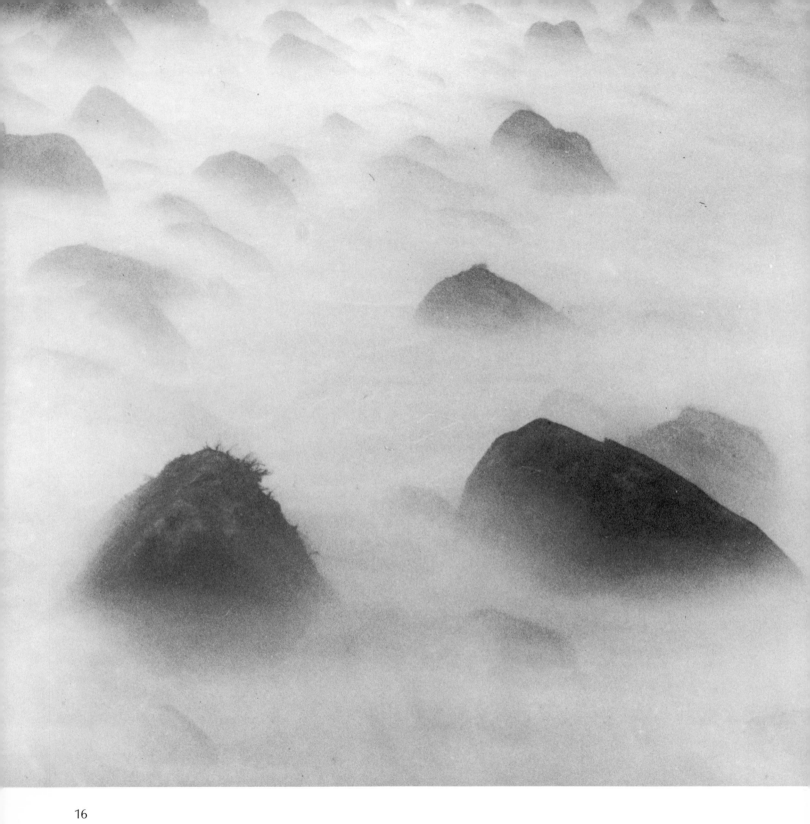

MICK CSAKY

Mick Csáky spent eight years at Art Schools studying painting, design, photography and film. He left the Royal College of Art, London, in 1971. His time is now divided between his family, directing documentary films for television and the cinema, and making multi-media contributions to exhibitions and museums of art, architecture and anthropology.

Experience is everything

In June 1974, during the preparation of this book, I felt it necessary to visit John Lilly, especially because of his work investigating the effects of sensory deprivation. I had read his startling book *The Centre of the Cyclone* which charts his penetrating explorations of his own consciousness – involving LSD, mysticism, several of the growth techniques and sensory deprivation. I was anxious to experience the effects of his sensory deprivation tanks, to test out for myself his theory that once the mind and senses have been released from their many environmental/survival chores, the mind is free to concentrate on the very creative and indeed exciting task of self-investigation. At dawn I drove up the Pacific coast to his home in Dekka Canyon, just north of Los Angeles, in the rugged folding hills of Malibu. We talked all morning. He quickly led me into complex and fundamental issues, concerning the nature of reality, of consciousness and God. . . . The early morning mist was burnt away by the dazzling Californian sun. I felt I was being tested by Dr Lilly. He was certainly not going to let me fool about in his sensory deprivation tanks, unless he felt I was approaching them in the right frame of mind. (It was only later that I learnt about the 'accidents' in the tanks, involving unsuitable yet eager explorers who had suffered disturbing experiences closed up in the dark.)

At length, quite casually, he offered me an hour in his latest tank – an eight-foot-diameter circular tank full of blood-temperature water which slowly revolved in total darkness. After a long relaxing shower I was instructed to cover my entire body with a heavy barrier cream to avoid being burnt by the thickly salted water in the tank. The salt was added to increase buoyancy. Next and somewhat ceremoniously I was led, in a towelled dressing-gown like a prize fighter, by Dr Lilly's wife Toni to the nearest hilltop. Thick white clouds now filled the canyon, like a Chinese watercolour. The warm wind felt good on my bare body under the dressing-gown. The dusty landscape resonated with life. The vibration of grasshoppers filled my ears. A simple wooden cabin perched on the top of the hill – more a lean-to than anything else. Although the wood was old, I could smell the resin in the bleached planks. Inside was the tank. It was a bulbous flying-saucer-shaped plastic object, connected to a supply unit which, Toni informed me, was pumping in oxygen and warmed water. She went on to explain that I would get most from my experience in the tank if I knew I was completely alone with myself. So, despite my obvious anxiety, she wished me luck and set off back down the steep hill, leaving me feeling very alone.

I walked thoughtfully round the tank and inspected the simple door and rumbling supply unit. It was cool in the deep shade of the cabin, too cool. I stepped back into the bright sunlight. Staring up at the heat of the sun, I shed my towelling garment. The dry wind was hot on my oily skin – but I felt cold. Impulsively, I stretched my body still closer to the sun and shouted 'Yes!' My voice was lost in the vastness of the landscape, and I did not hear myself. I shouted longer and louder, again and again, as if to confirm my own existence and the rightness of my actions.

As warmth flooded back into my body, my attention was brought abruptly back to the tank. The entrance door squeaked slowly open. With my heart pumping hard, I blinked and blinked as I peered into the shade, but my eyes were too full of sunshine. Then, out of the black square hole of the door, emerged a very wet, very naked woman with long black hair. She was young and brown all over – the first Red Indian I've ever seen in the flesh, I thought. She stepped silently into the sunlight beside me and stood very still, watching the water run off her body. My eyes explored her minutely with relaxed concentration. When her skin was dry with salty crystals she looked at me and, with apparent effort, focused her attention on me to nod and smile briefly. Saying nothing, she stepped forward and guided me to the tank. I lowered myself into the water and looked back for instructions. She raised her arms up, placed her legs well apart, shook out her hair and joined her fingers tightly behind her head. Then she bent her knees a little and arched her supple body backwards.

Breathing deeply, I followed along to find the position very stable in the buoyant water. Even with an arched back my nose and mouth stayed above the water, as it slowly spun me round. The revolving motion was caused by the pressure of many fine jets all round the circumference, which fed in freshly warmed water, at a slight angle. Staring up at the fibre-glass ceiling of the tank only three feet above me, I experienced a strong sensation of claustrophobia. At the end of one complete revolution I was staring directly up at my guide as she squatted in the doorway above my head. She nodded and simply said, 'I'll be back in one hour.' The door slammed shut. She was gone.

It was blacker than any black I had ever seen. The silence was louder than any silence. 'But I'm not ready yet!' I shouted, trying to sit up. I bumped my head sharply on the rough wall and fell back into the water. My mouth and nose stung sharply, my fingers groped helplessly for the door, but I could not tell whether I was reaching for the walls, the ceiling or the floor. The water was gone! I was floating in thin air! But as more salty water rushed into my eyes and nose I realized that it was still there, only as it was the same temperature as my body I could not feel it any longer. This brief act of reasoning calmed me down. I took several deep breaths and re-assembled myself into the correct floating position on my back again. Just like Leonardo's man in a circle, I thought, or Robert Fludd's Vitruvian figures. By will-power alone I dispelled my fears of drowning or suffocating, and gradually became accustomed to experiencing no body, no sound, nothing – a roaring silence.

Even though I was not really aware of being slowly revolved I could feel my centre of concentration, of being, shifting from my head to the turning point, the axis, of my body. As I continued to spin I felt my whole attention concentrating itself there, in my penis, my centre. Whether it was the cyclic motion of the tank or the vivid memory of my Indian guide's warm breasts pressing lightly against my body as I climbed into the tank I did not know, but my penis rose up and up – not an ordinary erection! It was the Eiffel Tower, the Empire State Building. As I arched my back further, sinking my head even deeper into the water, I felt my body matching the curve of the Earth's surface turning through space. My erection drew me up, like a moonshot from the ocean's floor, through thick wet clouds, through a fine dazzling mist. With grace and precision I orbited the Earth just once and came to rest in the blue sky high above Dekka Canyon, Malibu. Like a giant zeppelin, I thought, and laughed out loud. My mind flashed back into the tank. I had the strange sensation of soaring back and forth between my zeppelin form in the sky and my limp body floating in the tank, intercutting my rational attempts to explain what was going on in my mind with my desire to be transported by my daydreaming, my fantasy and imagination.

My body suddenly dissolved. I was falling down to earth in a cloud of raindrops. It was as clear and simple as a schoolbook diagram: the water is drawn up from the sea by the sun, and falls back as rain from the clouds into the sea or onto dry land. I fell softly onto the hard dry rock of the canyon and lay suspended in the red dust. Little by little my being seeped down further still, among the crevices in the rocks. Nothing could stop my movement as I slipped past brightly coloured fossils, past compacted strata of many rock forms, some glinting and crystalline.

I never felt the transition from hard to soft. One moment I was manoeuvring among atoms of granite, the next I was being carried along a subterranean river, rolling, turning and spinning. The river slowed down as I merged with the sea. I lay still and quiet and thought of nothing. The notion of time had completely left me.

My calm was broken by the increasing sensation of not being alone. My whole body, even my thinking, was being compressed and restricted. It was as though someone else was floating in the blackness alongside me. We kept the same slow cyclic tempo going, tumbling over each other alternately on top and below each other. With a startling rush of recognition I cried out 'John!' as I knew it was my twin brother John. We were floating together in the womb. The emotional impact of the encounter moved me greatly. I lay suspended like a jellyfish, with tears flowing freely.

At length I withdrew from this startling reunion to consider how my young son Leo must have felt floating all alone for so long in his mother's belly. Very soon I was Leo, floating in his mother's womb, in my wife Jean's womb, in my own mother's womb again, but this time all alone. The water stopped spinning me round. My body froze, passive with fear. My heartbeat was joined by a thunderous echo. The sides of the tank erupted inwards with unstoppable force against my fragile body. I slipped over their slimy surfaces as they closed upon me. As I resisted I was more tightly constricted. My lungs, my head, my entire body was being crushed alive. I was caught in a crack during an earthquake. I gasped for breath. Hot blood burst through the membrane of my body. The earth rumbled and groaned.

> *My mother groaned, my father wept*
> *Into the dangerous world I leapt*
> *Helpless, naked, piping loud,*
> *Like a fiend hid in a cloud.*

Something somewhere in me told me this was all an hallucination, yet I could not withdraw from its reality. I tried, with the desperation of a deep-sea diver without oxygen, to escape from the suffocating terror. I was rising fast, too fast, but it was the only way out. My mind blacked out as I rushed into a sunrise of spinning white light – too fast and too wild. I grabbed frantically for something to hang onto. I kicked wildly at the pain in my legs. A sharp sensation ran through my body. I kicked again and gasped sharply for breath. No air filled my lungs. I gasped again and again.

As quickly as I had entered the idea of being Leo in his mother's womb, I was out of it – floating in the darkness of the tank. My throat was sore and dry. The skin on my face tight with salt crystals. My ears roaring with the sound of my body's own metabolism. I was a child again, waking from a dream, calling out for his parents, but not heard. I laughed out loud at the ideas I was having. Leo, my son, laughed too – so loud in my ear that my body jerked sharply. I was with him, six or seven thousand miles away, rolling on the rough brown carpet of the bedroom in our flat in Bloomsbury. His wet lips bit against my cheek and ear as we laughed together. Jean was on the bed looking down at us and smiling. When she asked what was so funny I could not explain at first. Then I said, 'My God! It's true, like John Lilly said, all and everything that I imagine becomes real. Everything I am thinking of is becoming real in my mind, it is happening now.' Jean smiled quizzically and nodded sweetly. We both looked up together. Someone was knocking at the door. The knocking became more insistent. I blinked in the blackness. An unfamiliar voice called from far away, 'Are you OK?' With reluctant effort I answered, recognizing the Red Indian woman's voice. 'I'm going to open the door,' she said. My realities were flooded out by the sharp clear light. Even in the shade inside the cabin it was too bright. I was lying in a pale blue plastic tank of salty water, turning slowly round. The clear brown face stared at me as I must have stared at her. She was dressed now. I sat up, a little foolishly. She held out my dressing-gown, smiling. I clambered obediently out and let her wrap it gently round me. 'Fine time?' she inquired casually, but seeing my inability to find an appropriate answer, she simply nodded reassuringly and led off down the hill to the house. I wandered after her, in no hurry, stopping to stare closely at every little detail that caught my eyes: a piece of thistledown, a dead grasshopper, the dusty grit on the narrow path. . . .

Title page of Robert Fludd's *Utriusque Cosmi . . . Historia*, 1617. One of the images most vividly recalled by the author when John Lilly asked him to write down what he had experienced in the revolving sensory deprivation tank.

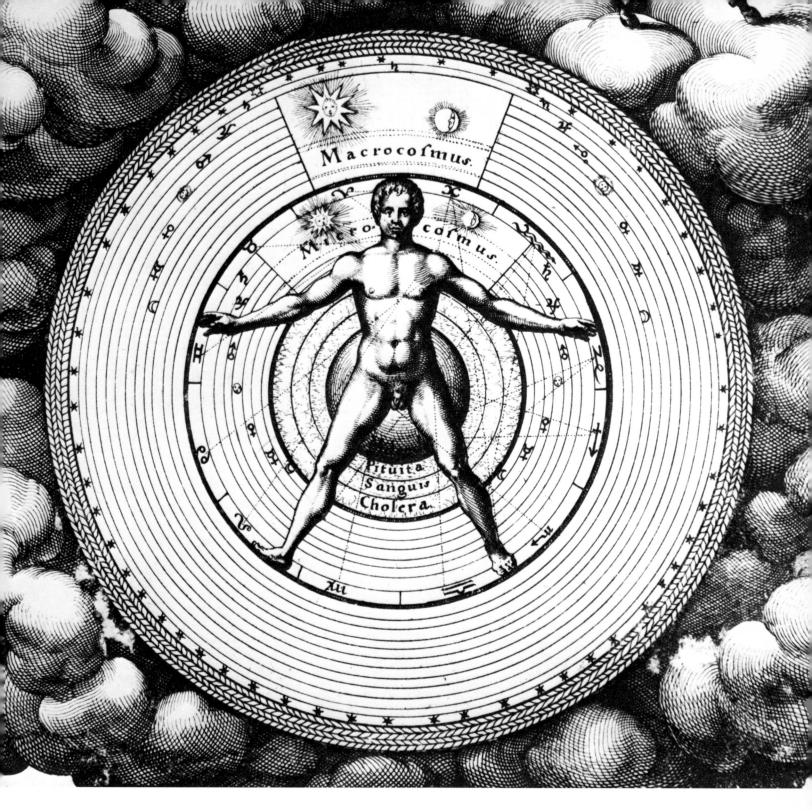

21

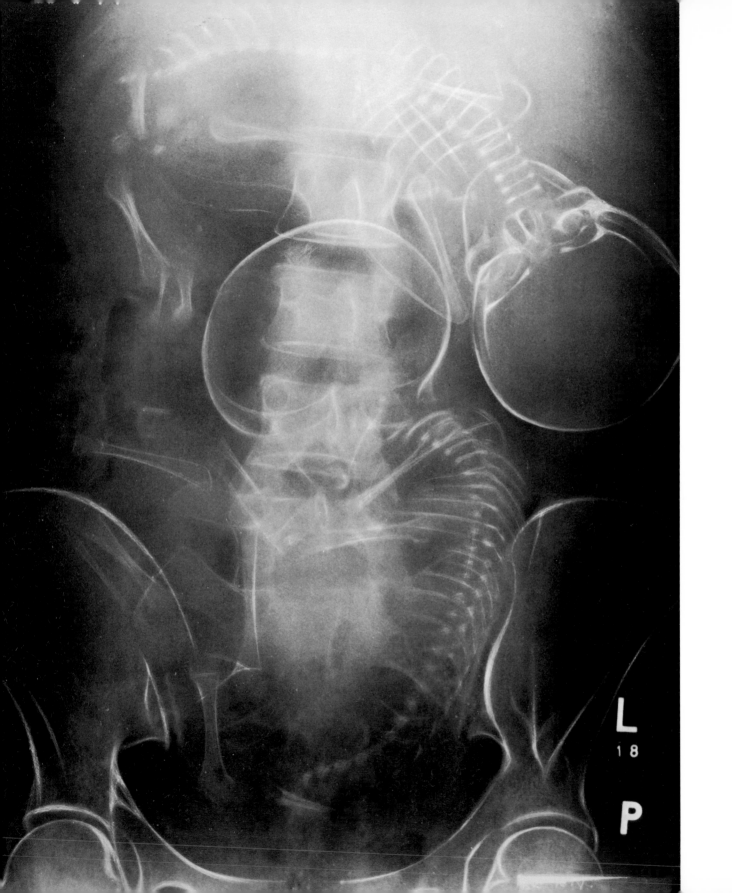

I did not sleep for the three days following. I did not seem to need to. Nearly four years later the impact of the experience is fresh in my mind. It was an experience that no amount of reading about, or indeed seeing films about, could ever repeat for me. It was an experience that was very relevant to this book, especially when I realized that it was going to be impossible to convey such important personal events to anyone with the vivid force with which I had experienced them. To put it another way: it is far more nourishing to eat the feast of life than simply to read the menu.

X-ray photograph revealing the author's twin children, who were conceived shortly after the tank experiences related in this chapter. The image bears a startling resemblance to the author's memory in the tank of floating in his own mother's womb with his twin brother John.

*Colour is a power
which directly influences
the soul. Colour is the
keyboard, the eyes are
the hammers, the soul
is the piano with many
strings. The artist is
the hand which plays,
touching one key or
another to cause vibration
in the soul. It is
therefore evident that
colour harmony must
rest only on a
corresponding vibration
in the human soul.*

Wassily Kandinsky

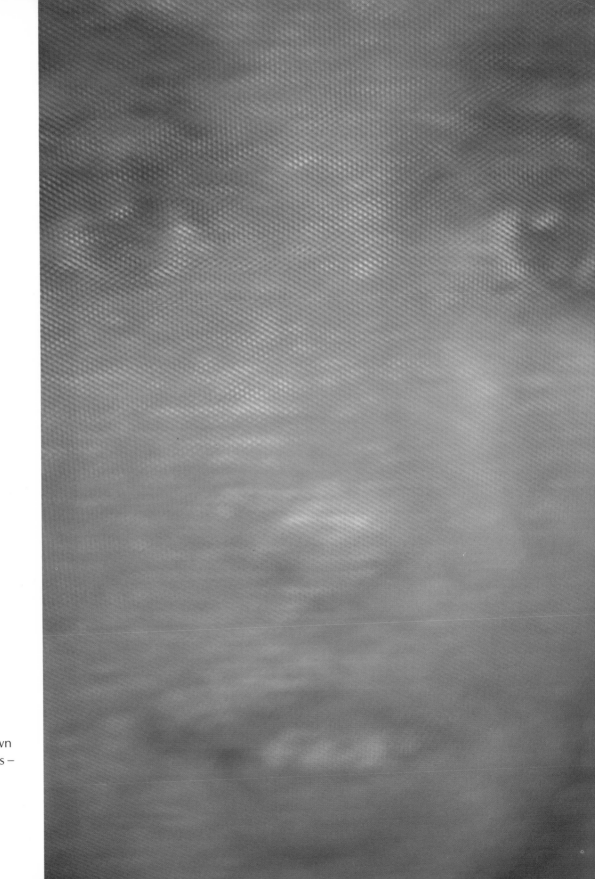

This close-up of a television
image breaks the picture down
to its component colour units –
the keys of the keyboard.

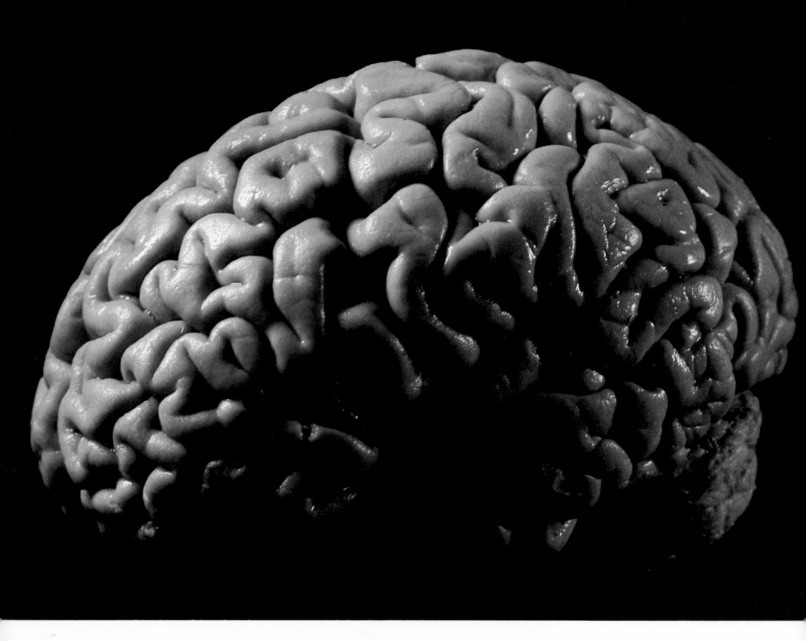

The intricate convolutions of the human brain increase the surface area to over 1000 square cm, and it is the outer 4 mm or so that are responsible for inquiry, foresight and creative ideas. Deeper within lie the sensory areas – touch and taste, sight and hearing.

'By comparison with our knowledge of the physical world we understand remarkably little about how we experience or perceive the world of things. Perhaps we know more about the interior of stars than the process going on in our heads which gives us feeling and knowledge.'

Richard Gregory

'The Raphaelesque Eclat'
by Salvador Dali

'Our body is a universe teeming with galaxies of worlds of its own, and a study of this is of much more import than a journey to the moon.'

Jean Cocteau

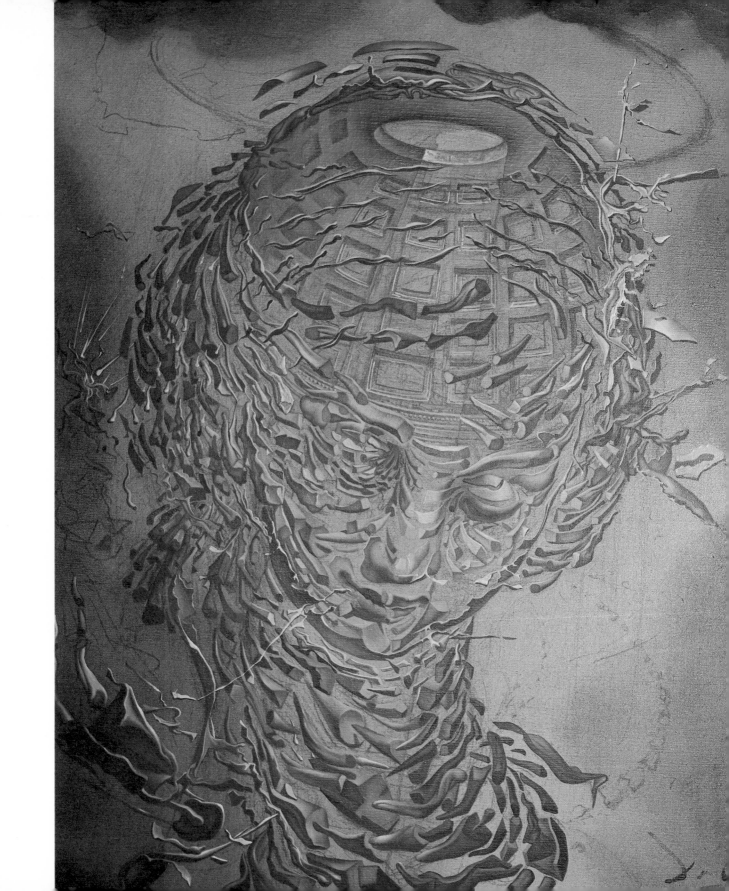

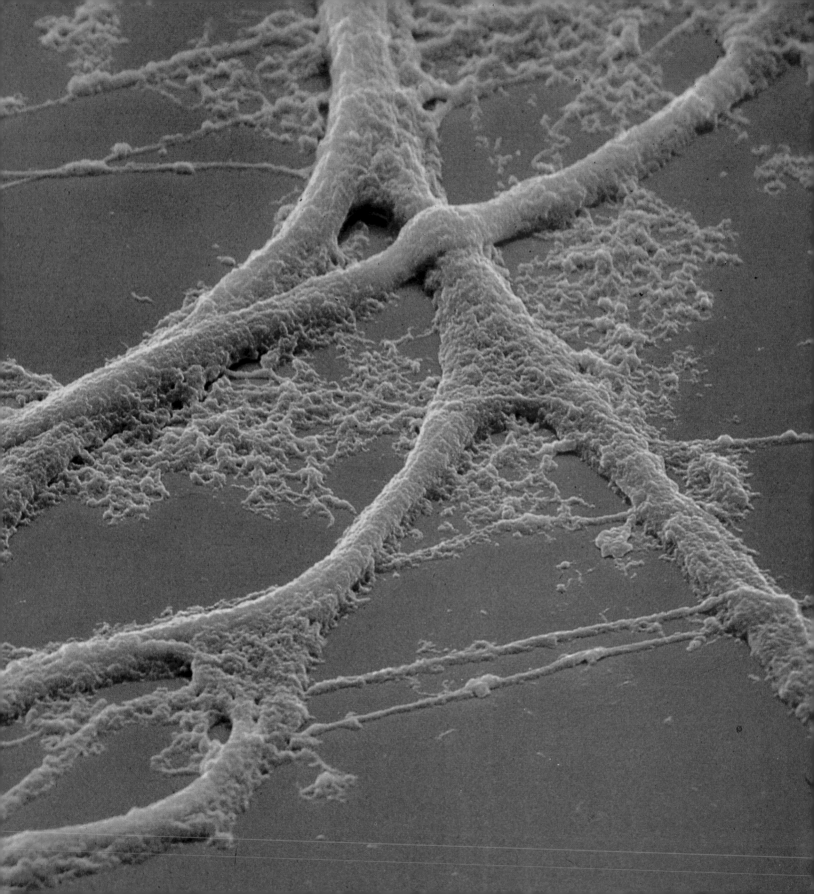

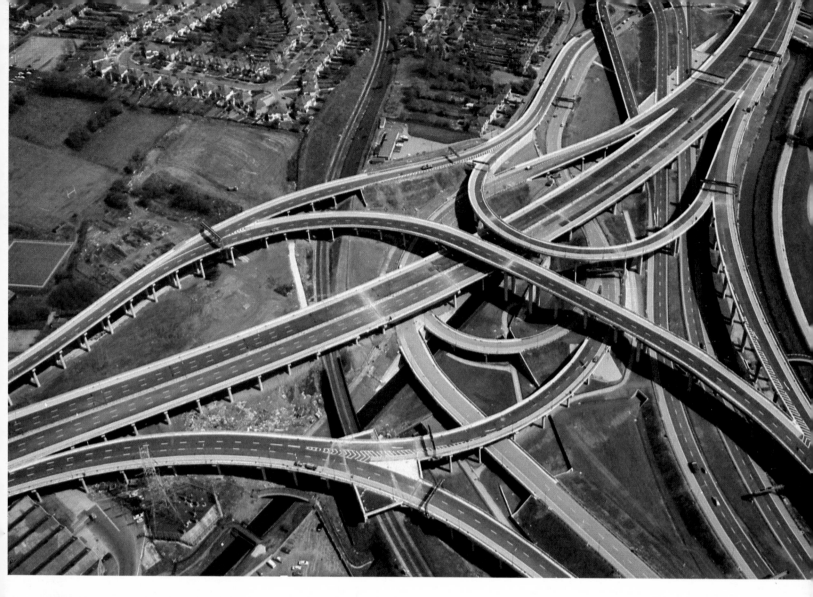

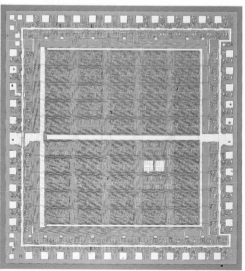

Magnified 150,000 times by the electron microscope, a group of nerve fibres and their junctions (synapses) bear an uncanny resemblance to a modern motorway junction (above, Gravelly Hill, Warwickshire, near Birmingham). Technology simulates nature also in the micro-circuits of modern electronics: the intricate but precisely designed labyrinth of impulse-paths shown here is actually little more than an eighth of an inch wide.

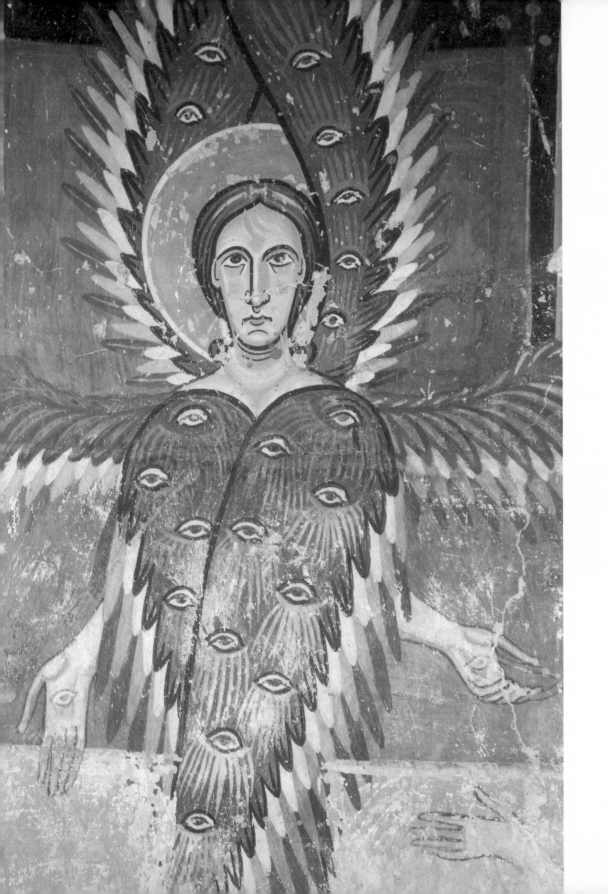

'If the doors of perception were cleansed men would see the world as it really is – infinite,' wrote Blake. But what is this perception? How do we 'see the world'? Through the eyes of mystics or of mortal men? The one is symbolized by an angel in a medieval Spanish fresco, the other by Lennart Nilsson's photograph taken through the iris of a human eye.

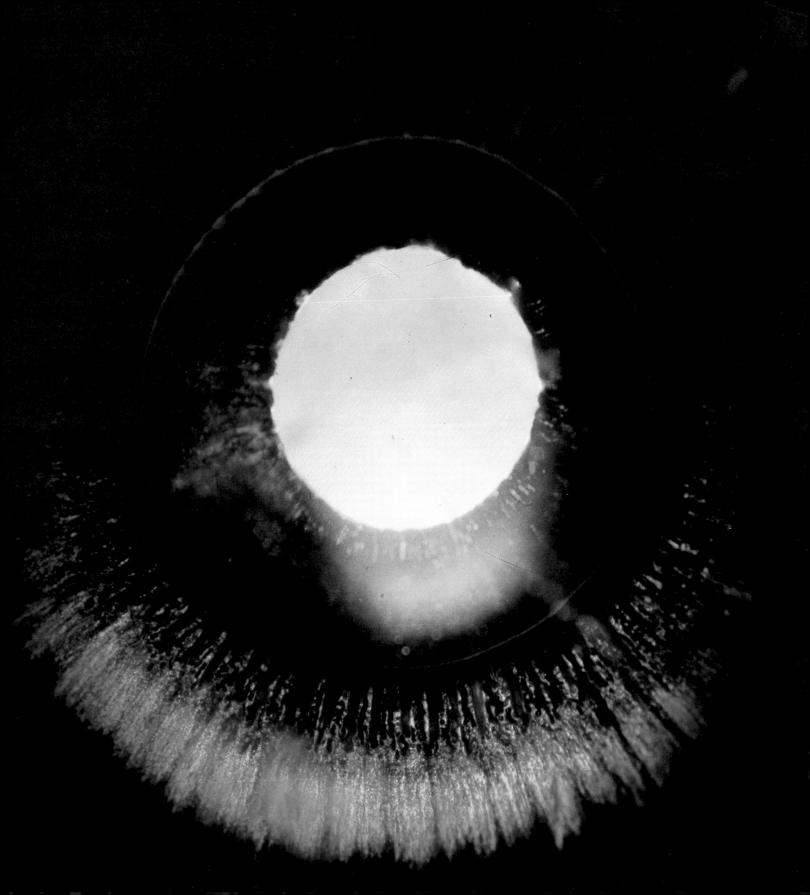

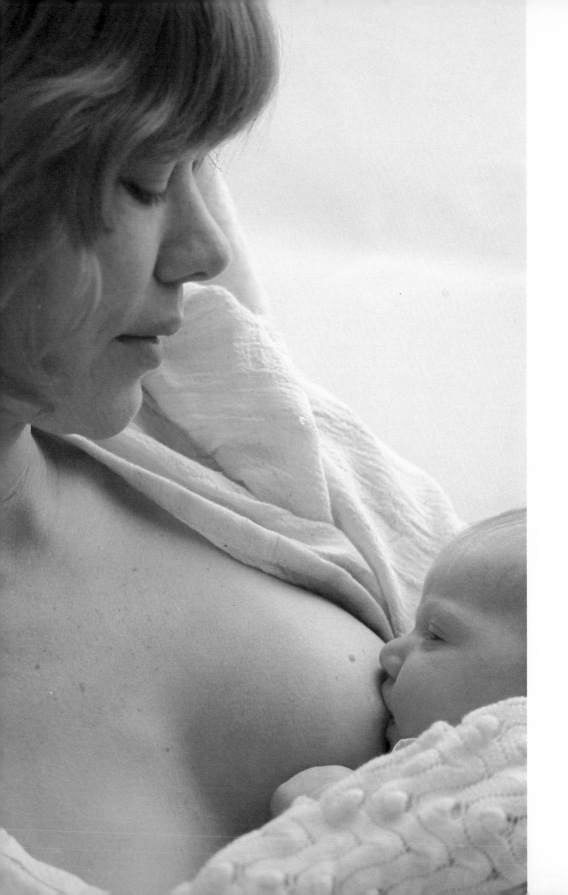

Blest the infant Babe
Nursed in his Mother's arms, who
　　　　　　　sinks to sleep,
Rocked on his Mother's breast; who
　　　　　　　with his soul
Drinks in the feelings of his Mother's
　　　　　　　eye!
For him in one dear Presence, there
　　　　　　　exists
A virtue which irradiates and exalts
Objects through widest intercourse of
　　　　　　　sense.
　　　　　　　Wordsworth

There is but a red rounded Moon
A fountain of white milk
For delight
The unobtainable Bliss
Has engulfed me
A precipice
Of light.
　　　　　　　Pattinattar

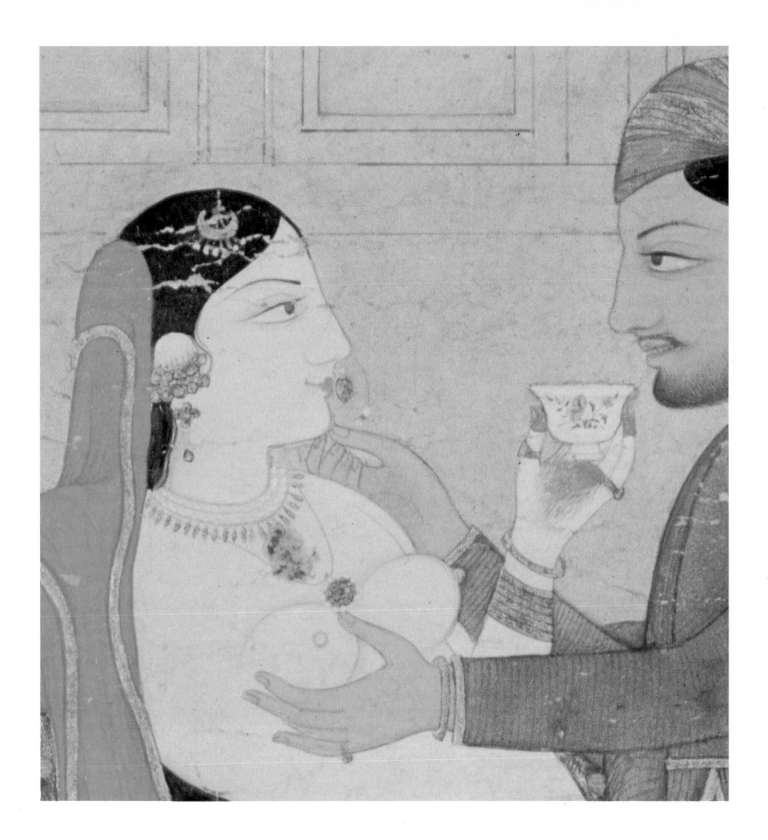

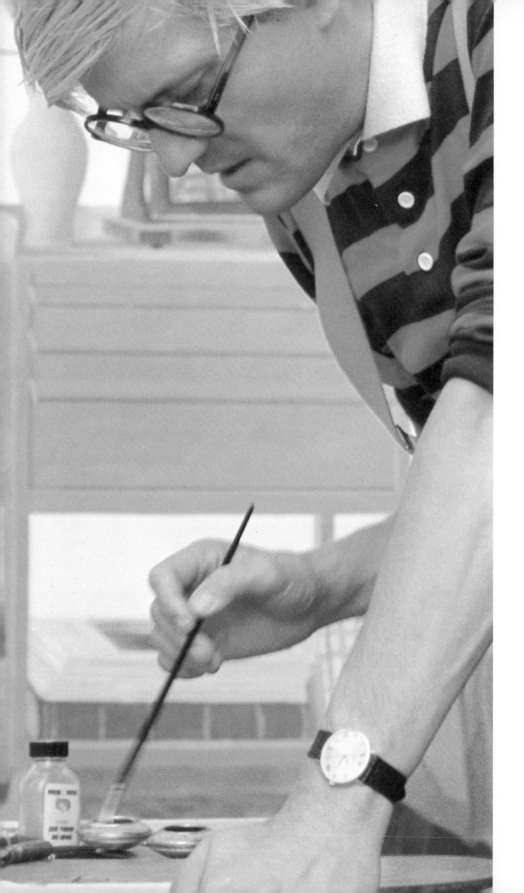

'I think it is good to follow the senses. It is good to trust your intuition, which of course not many people do; they think it is difficult. I thought it was very easy because I have always trusted mine, but I slowly realize that most people don't. That's all part of trusting your senses.'

David Hockney

'What does music really express? It's not about the sensations apprehended from the external world but about the intimations, intuitions, dreams, fantasies, emotions, the feelings within ourselves. … Why we want this nobody knows, but human beings certainly do need it as part of something for which I think we must use the word 'soul'. We want our souls to be nourished, and unless they are nourished we are dead.'

Michael Tippett

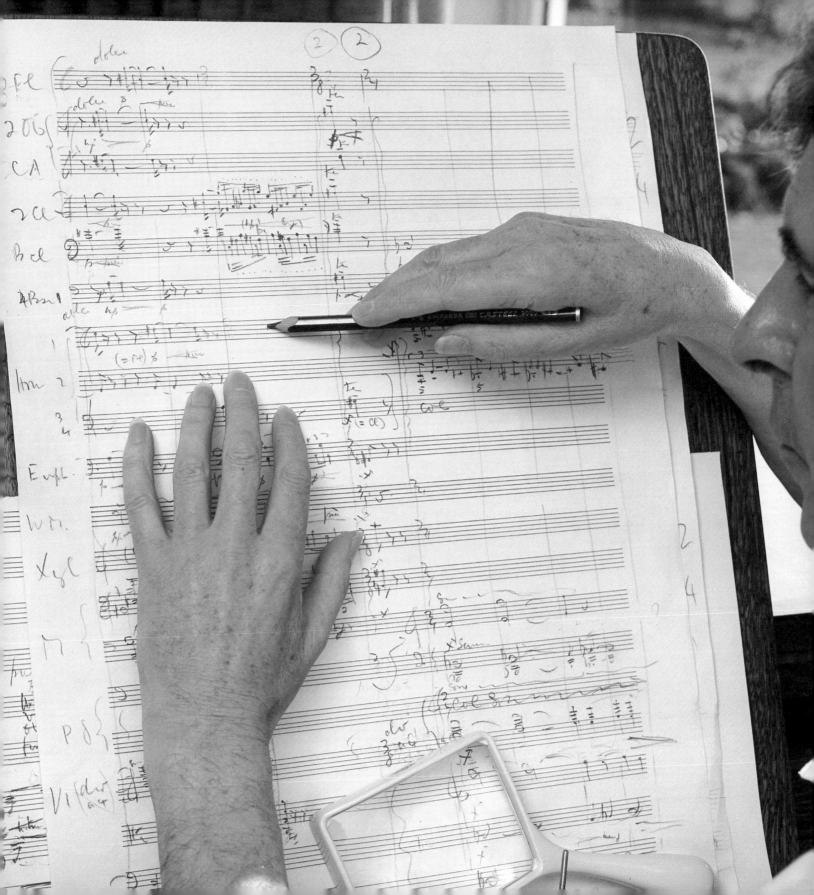

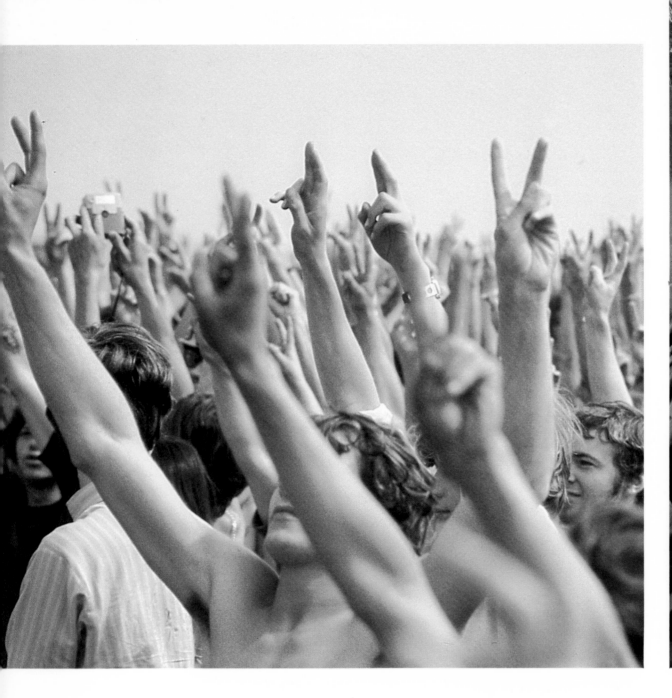
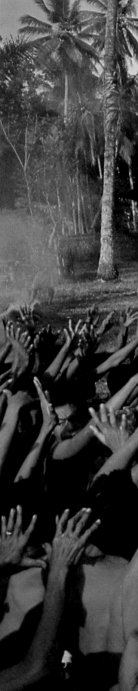

Equally at a pop festival or among Balinese worshippers the individual has entered a resonating tribal world in which the electronic extensions of everybody's nerves involve him deeply.

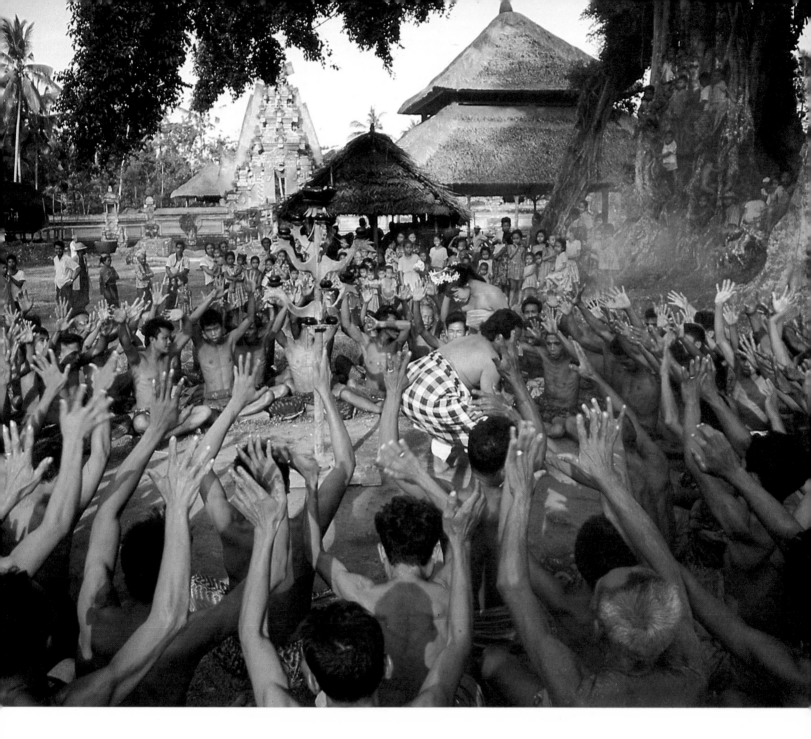

'People who can express emotions can more readily experience them. . . . In tribal
societies especially, perception or cognition is associated with, or immediately
followed by, an "emotion".'

Edmund Carpenter

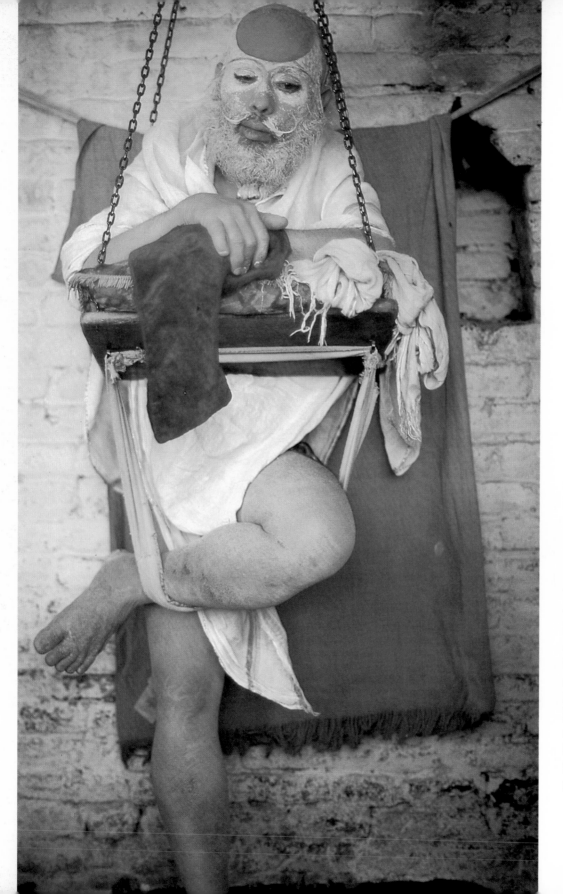

Two very different attitudes to the human body are presented here, illustrating diametric opposites of East and West. The Hindu holy man, photographed at the Shiva Ratri festival in Nepal, has balanced on one leg for seventeen years; ignoring and transcending physical pain, he has left the body behind in the inward-turned search for spiritual truth.

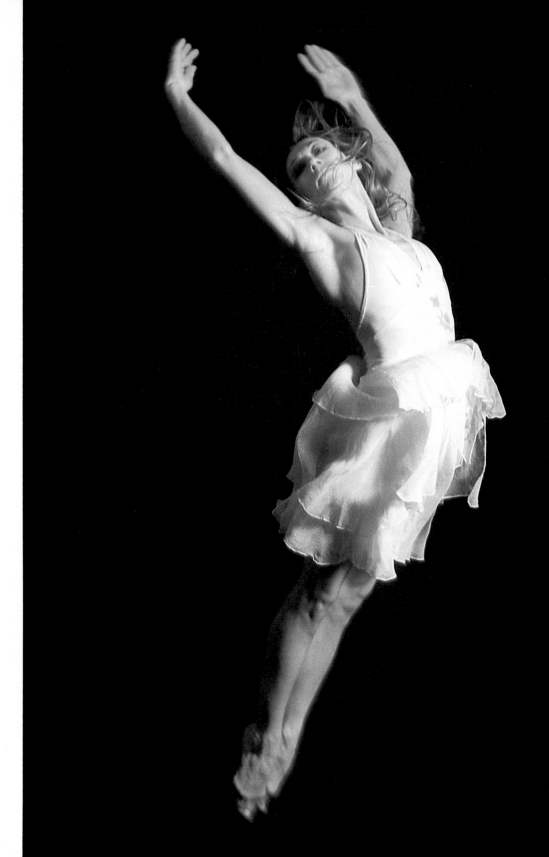

Linda Gibbs, of the
London Contemporary
Dance Theatre, employs
the body to express the
soaring of the human
spirit. The eastern goal is
spiritual attainment; the
western, artistic
expression by physical
means.

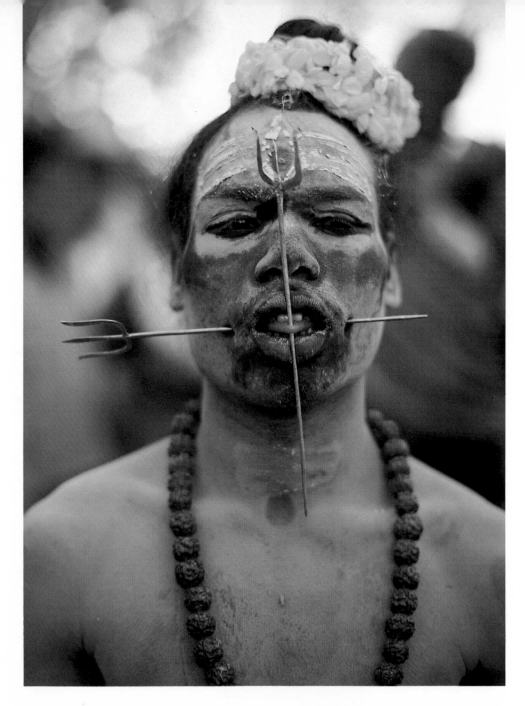

The self-mutilations of a *sadhu* and a
punk rock fan appear to have much in
common, but in fact the driving force
behind their actions could hardly
represent two more distant worlds.

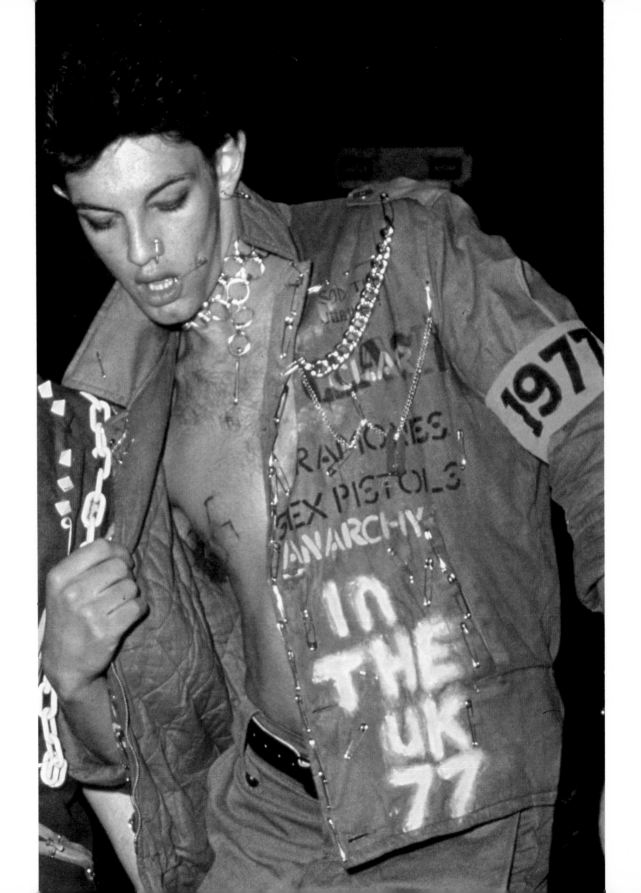

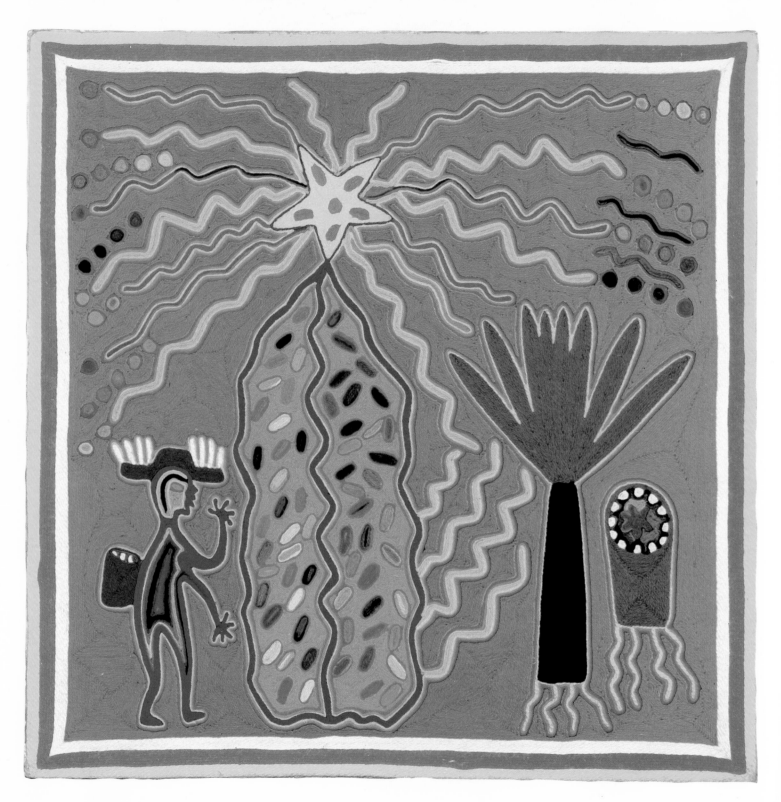

Our whole perception – and indeed understanding – of the world can be dramatically affected by the introduction of certain chemicals to the body, often in very small quantities. The picture opposite, made by a Huichol Indian in Mexico, shows a hallucinatory vision of the kind brought on by taking peyote. The Indian on the left is carrying a basket of freshly harvested peyote (the peyote cactus itself is shown in close-up at the right). In the centre of the picture is the vision that explodes in a blaze of colour and streaks and flashes of light.

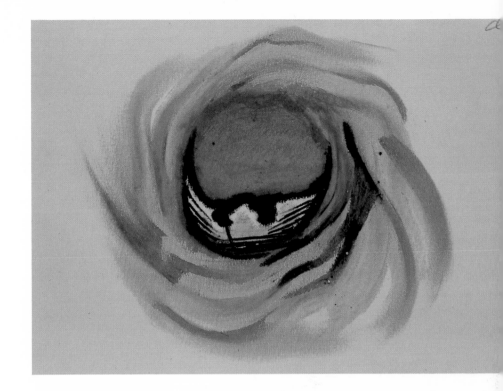

Doorknob seen at two different stages by an American artist while under the controlled influence of lysergic acid diethylamide (LSD) – 100 micrograms, taken by mouth.

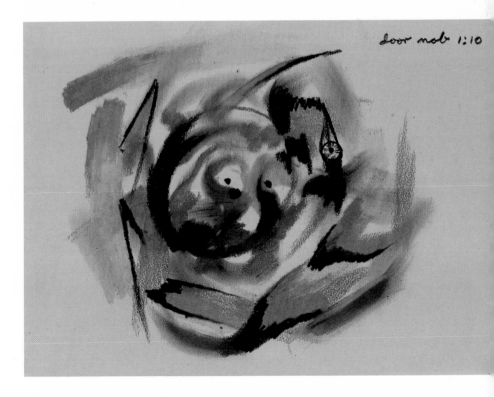

'We are men and our lot is to learn and to be hurled into inconceivable new worlds.'
'Are there any new worlds for us really?' I asked, half in jest.
'We have exhausted nothing, you fool,' he said imperatively. 'Seeing is for impeccable men. Temper your spirit now, become a warrior, learn to see, and then you'll know that there is no end to the new worlds for our vision.'
Carlos Castaneda

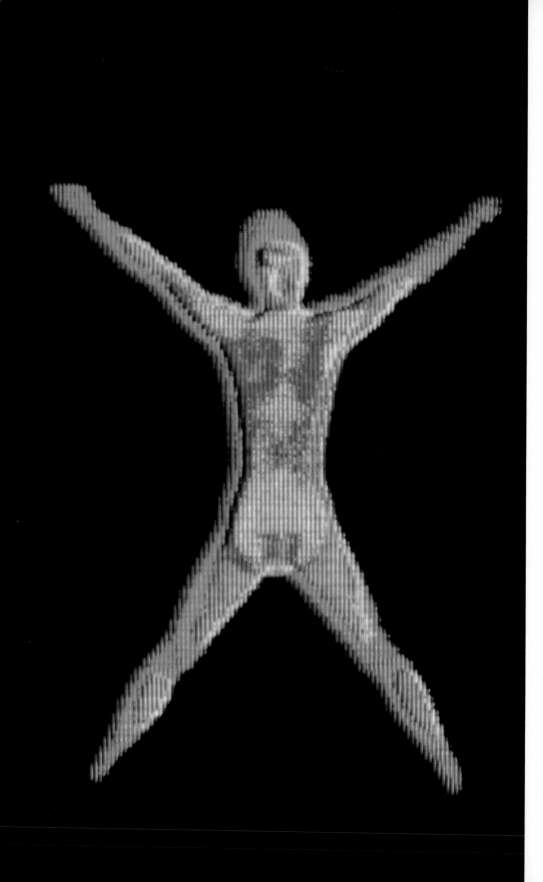

The human body gives off energy, and this can be quite easily detected and recorded scientifically. Infra-red radiation – which is to say heat – is shown by a thermograph camera, which translates temperature ranges into a colour code (left).

Less well known, and more spectacular in its imaging, is the high-frequency electrical discharge shown by Kirlian photography. This image (opposite) shows the fingertip of a person in a calm, resting state; illness, anger or mental disturbance can change this 'aura' dramatically, which suggests diagnostic possibilities.

Science thus seems to confer respectability on those 'sensitives' who claim to be able to see human auras. And could this be the origin of that common device in religious art, the halo?

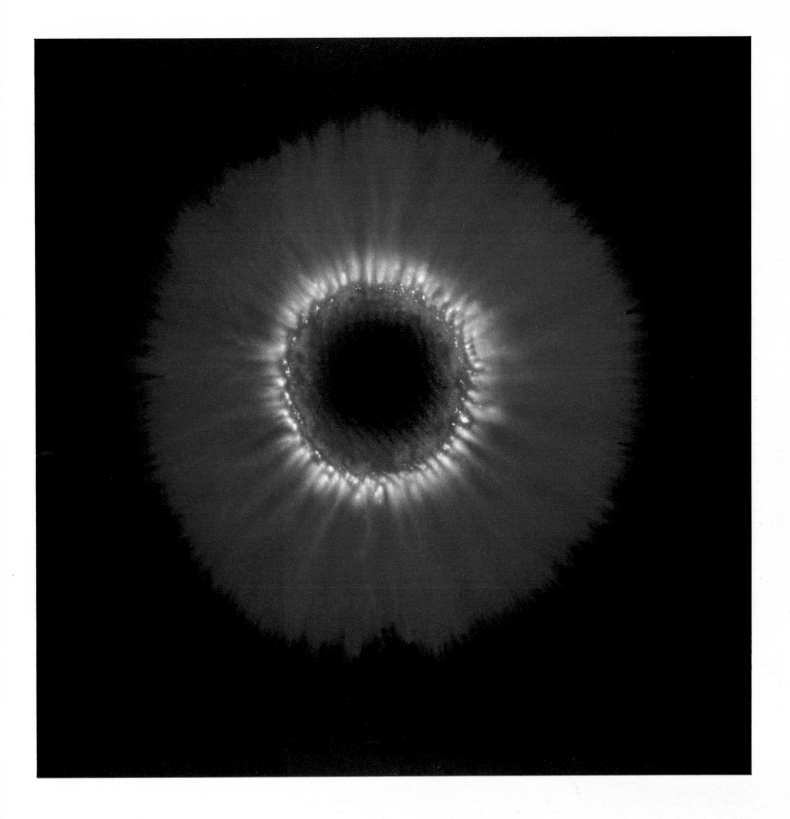

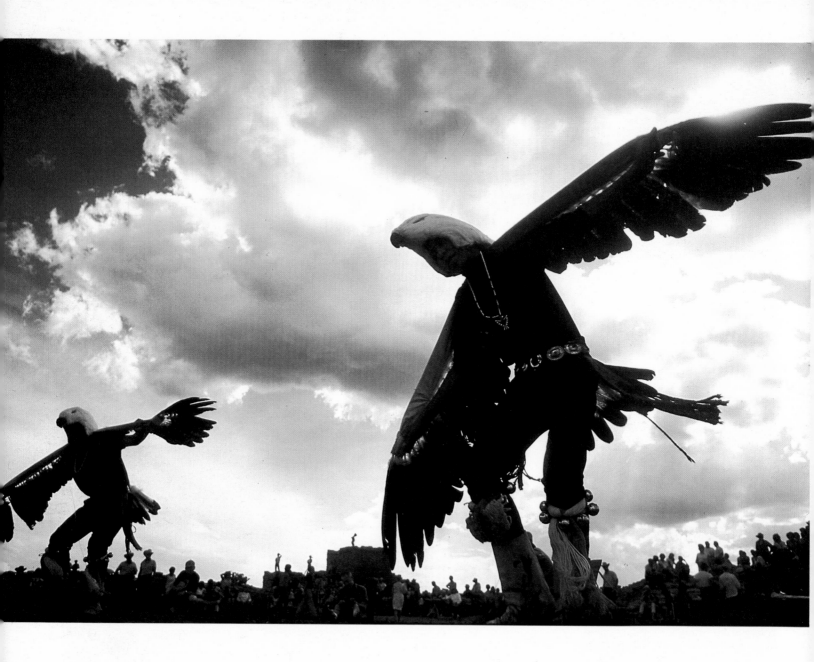

The Mexican bird-dancers strive for union with the natural world that surrounds and nurtures them. The men and women in the painting 'Focus' by Juan Genovès seem, on the other hand, to be not pursuing but fleeing – from what? From the world they have themselves created?

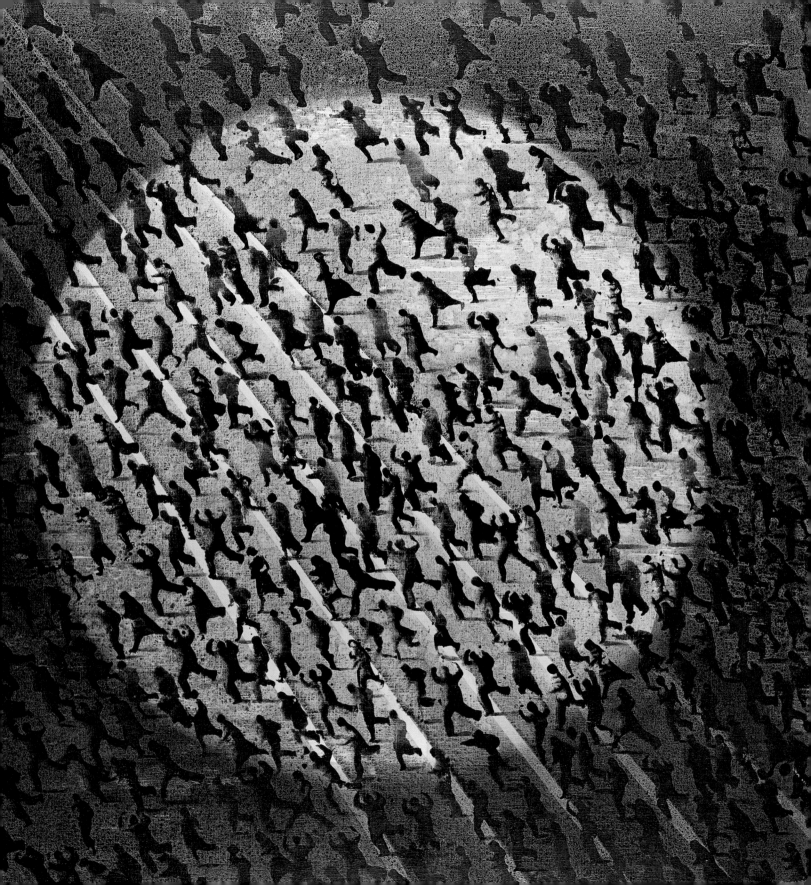

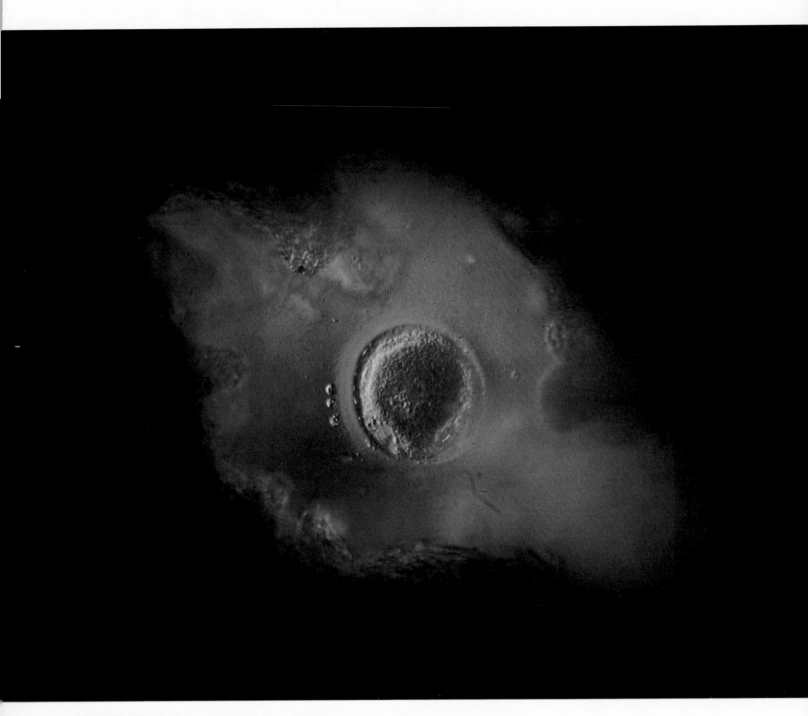

A human ovum, unfertilized, travelling down the Fallopian tube – first link in the chain of life.

I grew immersed in natural waters
like the mollusc in marine phosphorescence.
In me sounded the crusty salt
forming my singular skeleton.
How to explain—almost without
the blue and bitter movement of breathing,
one by one, the waves repeated
what I sensed and trembled with
until the salt and the spray formed me.
The scorn and desire of a wave,
the green rhythm which at its most secret
set up a tower of transparency.
The secret stayed and soon
I felt myself beating with it,
my voice growing with the water.

Pablo Neruda, 'Tides,'
translated by Alastair Reid

Drawing illustrating Paolo Mascagni's theory of the relationship between the tongue and the two halves of the brain.

PHYSIOLOGICAL FACTS:
how your senses work

Like the earth a hundred years ago, our mind still lies in darkest Africa, its unmapped Borneos and Amazonian basins. In relation to the fauna of these regions we are not yet zoologists, we are mere naturalists and collectors of specimens.

Aldous Huxley

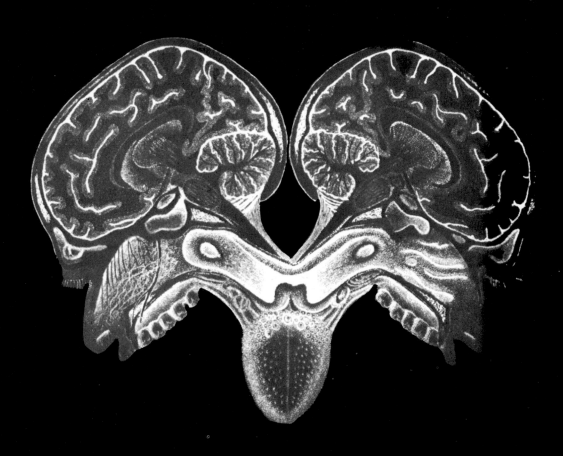

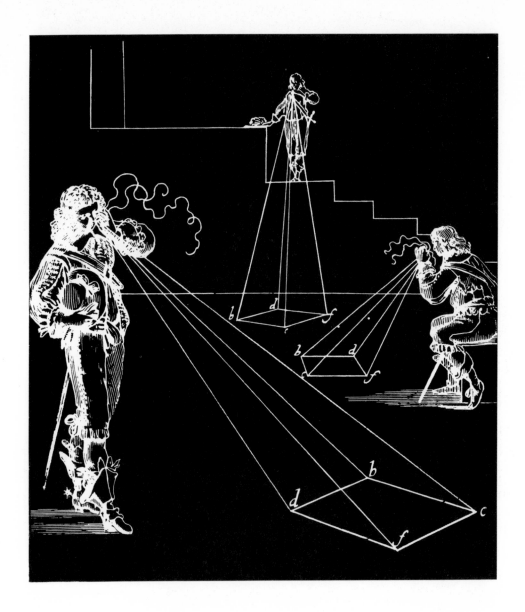

The convention of visual perspective demonstrated in a 17th-century drawing, placing each
viewer visibly at the centre of his world.

Opposite: a surreal study in perspective, photographed by Bill Brandt.

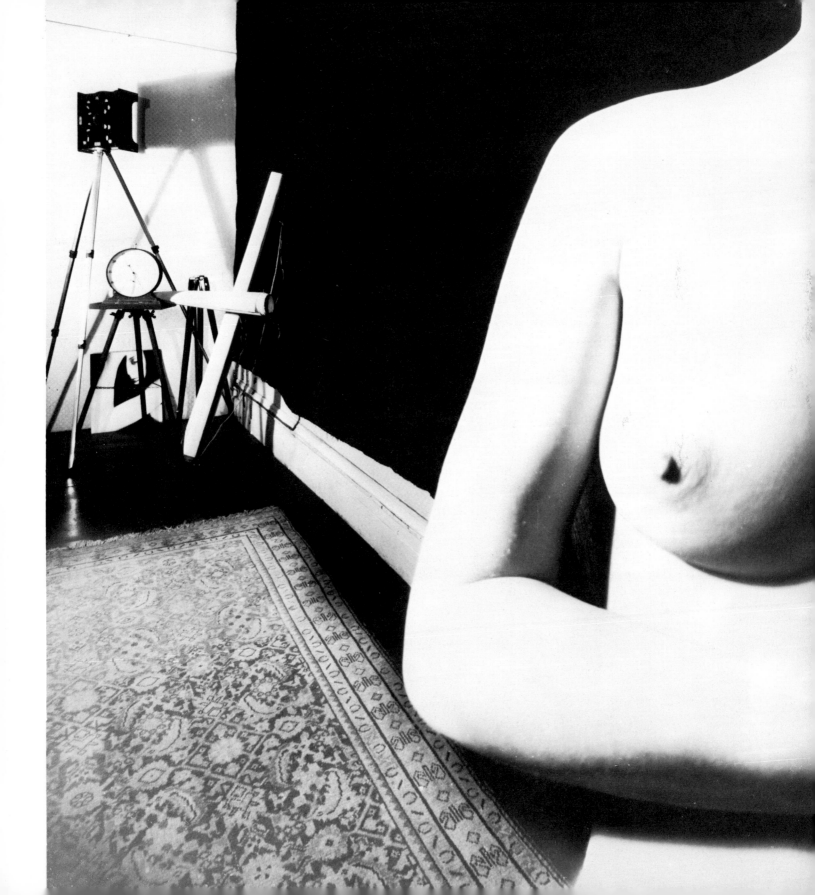

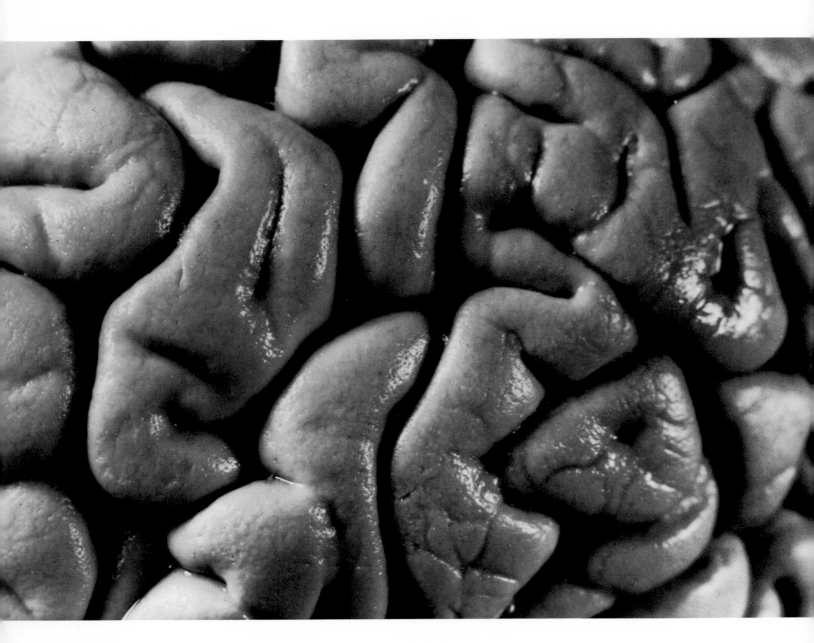

RICHARD L. GREGORY

Feeling the world by perception

Richard Gregory is Professor of Neuropsychology and Director of the Brain and Perception Laboratory at the University of Bristol, England. He has written several popular books on the subject of perception, including *The Intelligent Eye, Eye and Brain*, and *Concepts and Mechanisms of Perception*. He is currently compiling the *Oxford Companion of the Mind*.

Close-up photograph of the surface of the human brain.

Seeking food and mates and avoiding dangers are the first requirements for maintaining active life. For living in water, the sense of taste is most important of all because it directly monitors the chemical environment immediately necessary for survival. Touch and the related sense of pain are also of primary importance, as they monitor damage which, if continued, might rapidly cause death. Touch gives information only of objects in contact with the organism; but taste can allow distant food sources to be discovered by following intensity gradients. We may think of touch, of taste and of smell as *primary* senses, as they directly monitor conditions immediately necessary for survival. With the evolutionary separation of species into predators and prey, there was a growing need for information about more distant objects, especially threats and goals to be attained but distant in space and time.

All sensory information is ambiguous. Vibration in water may signal a dangerous predator; but the same vibration may be due to the harmless eddy of a gentle current. So even for a vibration sense it is a question of whether the signal is significant, or what its significance may be. Its significance depends on its origin – its source – which must be assumed or guessed. For touch and taste, however, there is not quite the same need to infer or to guess the origin of the sensation, for the chemical states they monitor are important in themselves. This is the most primitive and most direct kind of perception and knowledge, but it is extremely limited. An underwater vibration is a more subtle and less reliable source of knowledge, for it has to be 'read' to indicate something else, such as a predator or prey. The sense of vision is even less direct – and more ambiguous and more powerful. Vision is the sense most dependent on checks and calibrations from the more directly *monitoring* senses, which in their limited ways are more reliable through being less ambitious in reading rich realities from limited signals. The optical images of the eyes, by probing space, can for an intelligent brain also probe the future: to allow anticipation and strategic behaviour – freeing organisms from the tyranny of reflexes set off by stimuli, which limits primitive organisms to the here and now. There must have been an immense evolutionary pressure to extend perception into the future. Once events occur, it is too late to avoid or to control them. Threats and rewards are always in the future: it is this, I suggest, that led to the probing senses and to the development of large brains, to intelligence and the power to predict from observing sequences and discovering how the universe works. We see the beginnings of prediction even in plants. Plants respond to temperature, and other changes, which usually *precede* the spring, when they make their appearance. Their various stages of development are to be understood as triggered by conditions; but the triggering conditions are (in their simple cycling world of the seasons) predictive, so that they are prepared and ready for the next stage of the cycle. The reflexes of primitive animals (and our 'vegetative' reflexes) do much the same: they also serve to predict within simply repeating situations. As animals become through evolution more ambitious in their behaviour, they have to rely more and more on intelligent guessing, from their stored knowledge. This is the 'cognitive' aspect of perception: the intelligent deployment of knowledge.

Ancient stored knowledge is found in all reactive life forms. Even simple 'automatic' reflexes embody knowledge of the world and give some capacity for the simplest organisms to cope with common situations. This knowledge is not conscious.

It is often said that there are five senses – vision, hearing, touch, taste and smell – but in fact there are many more. Warmth and cold are signalled by receptors, and tickle is the ancient vibration sense vital for underwater creatures, for warning of danger and useful for signalling between mates. Then there are many senses indicating internal states, most obviously pain – of which there are several kinds – and also positions of the limbs and the tension of muscles. Not all of these senses reach consciousness: muscle tension, for example, is signalled by 'stretch receptors' rather like engineers' strain gauges; though highly important for the control of the body, they do not signal to the upper regions of the brain associated with consciousness. Vision, hearing and touch have clearly identified regions of brain devoted to elaborate mechanisms serving them. All the senses, whether or no they give sensation, or feeling, signal information of the outside world or of bodily states of their owner – be it to you or me, or some other creature very different from us, yet sharing the same world.

Primitive organisms have small, or even no, nervous systems. Their behaviour may be as limited as advancing or retreating according to the strength of signals at receptors. In this way they may follow gradients of a chemical concentration, or of temperature, or intensity of light with 'tropisms'. Tropisms, however, can be quite complicated: set by neural 'logic circuits' so that in some conditions a tropism is switched off, or switched from positive advancing to negative retreat. In even simple organisms, internal states are monitored in subtle ways to maintain metabolism; so senses have far more to do than appears from behaviour. This is so even for plants (which of course have no nervous system) for they have subtle detectors of gravity, humidity, and chemical senses for control of their green-blooded metabolism. Plant behaviour is indeed remarkable, from following the sun, responding to insects and even trapping them, to predicting the seasons. If they were quicker they might appear intelligent.

The eye, and ear, and other receivers of information are remarkably sensitive. The eye can respond to a flash of a few hundred quanta (the smallest unit of energy) and would be more sensitive still but for light lost in the media of the eye itself. The retinal receptors (the 'rods' and 'cones' which signal black-and-white and colour respectively) are sensitive to as little as one or two quanta – and so they have the maximum possible theoretical sensitivity. The ear also is as sensitive as it could be. It has been calculated that in the cochlea, where by a process not fully understood frequencies of air vibrations are separated spatially around its spiral structure, the basilar membrane vibrates with an amplitude half the diameter of a hydrogen atom at the faintest sound we can hear. By touch, we can feel ridges less than a thousandth of an inch in height, and the vibration sense of the skin is even more delicate. The range of intensities over which the senses work is also remarkable: the eye functions (with dark/light adaptation) over a range of a million to one intensity units, and will discriminate differences of a few per cent in intensity over most of this enormous range.

The images in the eyes do not enter the brain. Their patterns are transmitted down a bundle of nerve fibres, at about the speed of sound, by pulses of electricity giving coded messages. The basic code is: increasing frequency of pulses with increasing intensity of light. This long and complicated chain of events gives a very different notion of perception from the direct immediate knowledge we *seem* to have when we open our eyes and see the world around us. The brain has the task of reconstituting – or creating its own – reality from these pulse-coded signals which are its only messages from the outside world. When we experience colour, movement, sound, touch or smell, all that our brains receive are these chains of electrical pulses running down the millions of nerve fibres from the receptors of the various senses. The brain decodes, or 'reads', these patterns of pulses to give sensation and perception, but the signals are of no use until they are processed and read as messages.

There is an important analogy here to signals from scientific instruments. Signals of any kind are useless until they are processed to give data. Data are not physical, in the usual sense of the word, for data are given by reading and interpreting signals as symbols. This cannot be done with any instrument in the range of the physical sciences. An oscilloscope can show the signals in a nerve, but it cannot tell what the information is, or how much is being transmitted. And it certainly cannot indicate the information of *no* signals! We may recognize something from a *surprising absence* of signals. When signals or their absence are *surprising* they convey *information*. To estimate the amount of information conveyed we need to know how surprising – how unlikely – is the message or its absence. Perception is generally a matter of deciding between alternatives. The significance of alternatives is what makes perception essentially different from the physical world. The seventeenth-century physicists were concerned with what *happens* in given situations; but perception is continually concerned with what *might* happen. Perception does not merely signal what is, it generates alternative hypotheses of what might be. These hypotheses are predictive – for decisions, to be useful and have survival value, must be aimed at the future. In unusual situations – or if false assumptions are accepted – such procedures could generate errors in perception much as errors occur in science when inappropriate procedures, or false assumptions or premises, are adopted. This can happen at all stages of scientific observation, including deriving data from the signals of instruments by statistical methods. Indeed, the methods of science and the processes by which the nervous system gives us perceptual knowledge could be very similar. We may go further, to suggest that *perceptions are hypotheses of reality*. Some are no doubt true; but many (as in science) are more or less incorrect.

In some conditions a wrong alternative is accepted: then we have an illusion or an hallucination. Hallucinations are total departures from reality; illusions are discrepancies from reality – so neither are within physics. There are many kinds of illusions, and they can tell us a lot about perception. This becomes a technical and tricky business, but the following classification of illusions may help:

1   *Ambiguities*: such as the Necker cube, and the figure and figure/ground ambiguity of the Rubin figures (below).
2   *Distortions*: such as the 'café wall', the Zollner and Orbison figures (opposite).
3   *Paradoxes*: such as the Penrose impossible triangle figure, and other 'impossible objects' which exist in three dimensions but appear impossible from certain points of view (overleaf).

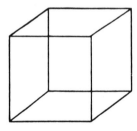

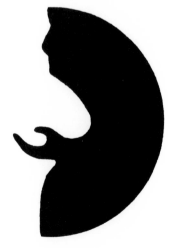

Ambiguities: two equally valid interpretations can be made, and we cannot be sure which is right. In the Necker cube, which square face is the nearer? Does the Rubin figure portray a face (white) or an old beggar woman (black)?

58

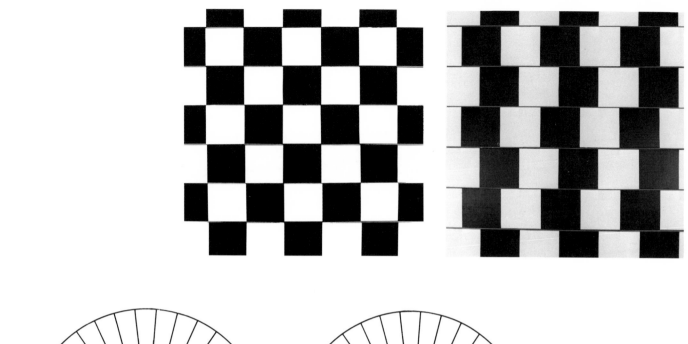

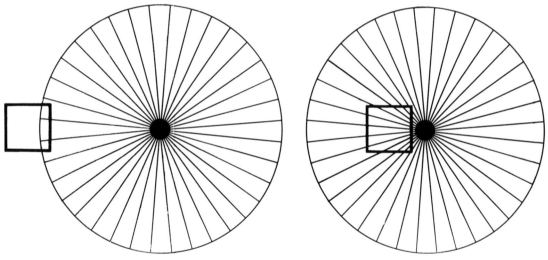

Distortions: in the 'café wall' illusion, when
alternate rows are displaced, the lines between
seem no longer parallel; in the centre is an
Orbison figure, in which the square seems
distorted when placed over converging radii; in
the Zollner figure the long oblique lines are
actually parallel.

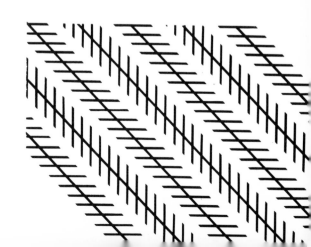

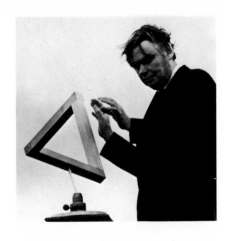

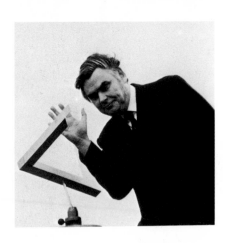

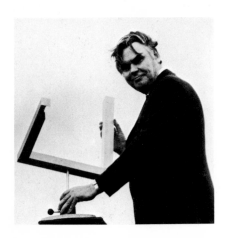

Hypotheses are very different from reality even when they are true. They are different because they are *descriptions*, or *explanations*, rather than copies. Further, there is an endless number of possible hypotheses for any event or situation, though some will be more useful, appropriate, adequate, or true than others. It is always a question which is the best hypothesis. The number of alternatives to choose from is – for science or for perceptions – limited only by imagination. This notion of selecting between alternative hypotheses follows from the concept of perception and science as being active hypothesis generators. It leads to the recent technical account of information as selecting between alternatives. This account of information was developed by C. E. Shannon, of the Bell Telephone Laboratories, and has made it possible to quantify and measure information in communication channels and computers. Unfortunately, though, it is not very helpful as a measure for brains, because we do not know how many alternatives we have to choose from, even for the simplest skill.

Each of the senses has its own kind of *receptors* which convert patterns of physical energy from the external world (times internal changes from within the organism) into the action-potential signals of nerves; but sensations are not simply related to the channels. For colour vision there are three channels (sensitive to red, green and blue light respectively) but colours as we see them are *mixtures* of these. Yellow appears as a simple colour but it is always given by a mixture of 'red' and 'green' signals. In general, sensations which seem to be simple or primary are not given by particularly simple physiological mechanisms. This very likely applies to that most basic sensation – pain – though how pain is signalled remains mysterious. It is particularly odd that pain is never elicited by direct electrical stimulation of any regions of the brain (during brain operations with conscious patients), though the other sensations are readily aroused in this way.

How are we – as observers – related to the world? The key discovery was made at the end of the tenth century by an Arabic scholar, Alhazan, who put visual perception into a clear relation with the physical world by inventing the *camera obscura*. This projects the world as an image on a screen. The principle is now so familiar, from slide projectors and cameras, that it may not look important or revolutionary, or least of all of philosophical significance. Its implications are still not fully realized even by some writers on perception. Alhazan, and later the astronomer Kepler, realized that the world is projected into the eye as an image, so that we do not have *direct* visual knowledge of the external world. We are connected visually to the physical world by a tenuous link of light-giving images very different from the objects we see and very different also from our perceptions. With the advance of the physical sciences, mathematical accounts of the universe threaten what we accept as knowledge by perception.

Physics took off from a few simple experiments in the seventeenth century, notably by Galileo, which gave insight into the kinds of things worth investigating and describing in detail, to flower in Newton's account a generation later.

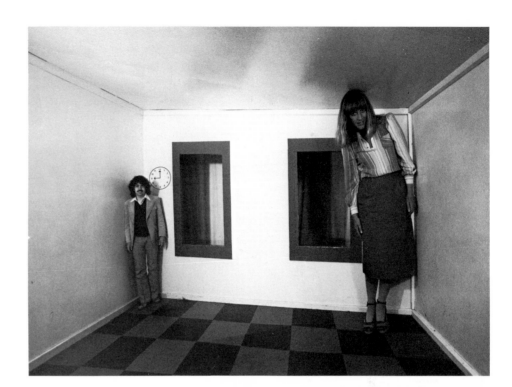

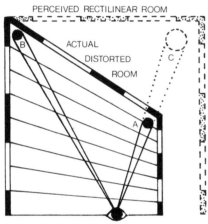

PERCEIVED RECTILINEAR ROOM

B

ACTUAL

DISTORTED

ROOM

C

A

PEEP-HOLE

Paradoxes: Professor Gregory (*opposite*) with the Penrose 'impossible triangle'. The Ames room (*right*) is deliberately designed (as the diagram shows) to counteract – when seen from one critical viewpoint – the converging lines of perspective. The room looks conventionally rectangular, while the human figures, which are actually the same height, look odd.

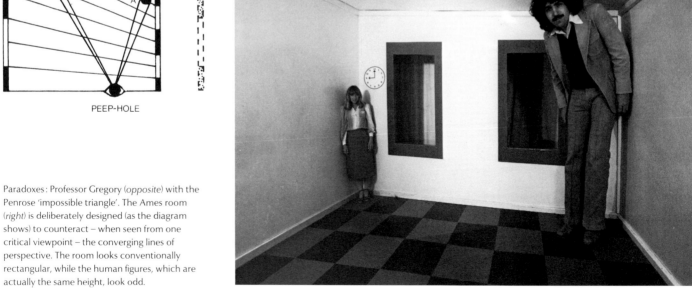

Astronomy gave essential keys for understanding the physical world, and for predicting and controlling a far wider range of events and situations than the brain unaided by science could achieve. The success of Newton's mathematical account of the universe was, however, bought at the cost of leaving out the observer. Science very largely ceased to care about why things appear to us coloured, hard, beautiful, or frightening.

This rejection of how things *look* in favour of how they must *be* to give simple mathematical descriptions, started with the Copernican switch of thought, from the sun moving round the earth (as we see it) to the earth moving round the sun. This was mind-jolting, running against what we seem to know directly by experience from the senses. The sun is *seen* to move across the sky, the earth *feels* stationary; such scientific insights came from abandoning sight and feel. With the new insights of science our most trusted sources of knowledge as well as our strongest beliefs became suspect and sometimes trivial. Lapse into total triviality of feeling was avoided by the artists; but they too suffered from science's rejection of experience as representing important or deep truth. The *sensations* of colours were not at all explained. How we see remained mysterious and was seldom questioned. The physical sciences went from one triumph to the next, to transform the way we live and understand, but left us as observers and knowers almost entirely out of account. The unprecedented success of Galileo and Newton demoted sensation and feeling, leading to the twentieth-century psychology of Behaviourism, which altogether denied feeling and consciousness.

Newton, however, did investigate the physics of colour, showing that all the colours of the spectrum (which was already known) produced by a glass prism are contained in white light. He was clear that light is not itself coloured, writing (*Opticks*, 160):

> The homogenial light rays which appear red, or rather make objects appear so, I shall call rubric or red-making: those which make objects appear yellow, green, blue or violet, I call yellow-making, green-making, blue-making, violet-making, and so of the rest....

Of coloured light he said: 'In them there is nothing else than a certain power and disposition to stir up the sensation of that colour.' He also allowed that the sensations of colours could occur without light:

> ... they appear sometimes by other causes, as when by the power of phantasy we see colours in a dream, or a madman sees things before him which are not there... or we see colours like the eye of a peacock's feather by pressing our eyes in either corner whilst we look the other way.

This was a contradiction of the notion that all the phenomena of light and colour could be put into physics, without reference to the observer as in a way separate, which Newton (frankly rather tamely) resolved in this way: 'Where these and such like causes interpose not, the colour answers to the sort or sorts of rays whereof the light consists.' This is very far from satisfactory, as Newton must have realized.

It is important to realize the remarkable power of brains to make highly efficient use of limited sensory information. In this, perception is like science, which also builds powerful predictive hypotheses from limited data given by the signals of transducers monitoring events. It is all too easy to see 'paranormal' influences when the power of 'normal' processes is under-appreciated. This same mistake can also produce such statements as: 'We should develop the senses to increase our experience and understanding.' The fact is that we have discovered magnetism, though we have no sense for detecting magnetic fields (while some other organisms do have such a sense) and in general we appreciate far more than we can sense. This may be an 'intellectualist' point to make but I believe, from what we know of the immense contribution of knowledge to what is signalled by the senses, that it is justified. What is important is not so much what we feel *as signalled*, but rather what significance we can attach to the limited signals of the senses by what we know. Knowledge enriches sensory signals to make what we feel interesting. Even this is an understatement, for sensations are themselves enriched and modified in many ways by knowledge. One might imagine that the sensation of a lifted weight is physiologically simple, signalled directly from the stretch receptors of the muscles. But the sensation of weight is affected by our knowledge of the *probable* weight of the object before it is lifted. This we know beyond doubt, for a *small* weight is sensed as *heavier* than a larger object of the same scale weight. This can easily be checked in a kitchen experiment with tins of different sizes filled with, say, sugar to make pairs of different-sized tins equal in scale weight. They will *feel* very different though they are the same weight. The *feeling* of weight increases with the *surprise* that the signalled weight differs from the expected weight. We feel it as heavier when it is expected to be lighter, smaller objects generally being lighter than larger objects. This same kind of situation holds for very many illusions – which are therefore indications of the power of knowledge (sometimes false) to affect how we feel.

The development and use of generalized knowledge became necessary as reflexes became inadequate. There are, however, still theories of psychology whose concepts are limited to reflex stimulus-response mechanisms; but their inadequacy should be clear from the importance of prediction. The biological significance of prediction for survival can hardly be exaggerated. This indeed provides rather strong evidence *against* 'paranormal' predictive powers – for if they existed at all surely they would be far better developed and so more clearly in evidence than they seem to be. There is still, after many years of arduous research, no clearly acceptable evidence for precognitive powers of prediction based on sources of information not available to the known senses. Decision-making may be done by informal procedures or may be rigorous. We are only beginning to understand the procedures through which neural signals become useful data, and how these sensory data are used to give decisions for perception. When the probabilities of alternatives are nearly balanced, perception is ambiguous, with spontaneous changes taking place though the pattern of stimulation is unchanging. Such phenomena are highly revealing for appreciating some of the more subtle processes of perception.

Sensory signals are so limited it is little short of miraculous that perception as we know it is possible. We act not merely on *signals* from the senses, but even more on *knowledge* of objects and situations. Sensory signals are hopelessly inadequate for giving control of the behaviour of organisms directly. Sensory signals arrive too late, they are intermittent, and they are very often but indirectly related to situations requiring action. Most likely it was the limitations of sensory signals that forced organisms to develop sophisticated perception, from the earlier basis of stimulus-response mechanisms giving the primitive reflexes. Perception required the development of knowledge of the world to make effective use of limited sensory data. We are not conscious of what must be almost incredibly elaborate data-handling processes giving rise to perception from signals and data from the past stored in the brain. Recent attempts to programme computers with television camera eyes to recognize objects shows how sophisticated these processes must be for making the required decisions.

Do computers have consciousness? If they should come to perform much as we perform perceptually, then we have a simple choice to make. We must either say that consciousness is not important for perception, or that computers displaying human-like perception are conscious. If we fail to make computers which can behave as we behave, our technological failure may provide evidence for our uniqueness. If we succeed, we may either say that consciousness is not causally important, or that consciousness is not restricted to brains but can be given by electronic circuits. So it seems that the development of artificial intelligence and artificial perception in machines is a route for pursuing this ancient philosophical question. If we succeed, we should discover the significance and causal importance of feelings. If we should fail in interesting ways, the problem of consciousness may appear not as metaphysics but as metatechnology. For the present, we have neither succeeded nor convincingly failed: so that we cannot yet give a biological reason from computer research for why we feel the world by perception.

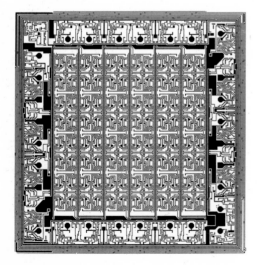

Opposite: Jean Cocteau's illustration of heightened sensory awareness, from his book *Opium*.

PSYCHOLOGICAL VARIETY:
interpreting the world through your senses

The world today hangs by a thin thread, and that thread is the psyche of man.

C. G. Jung

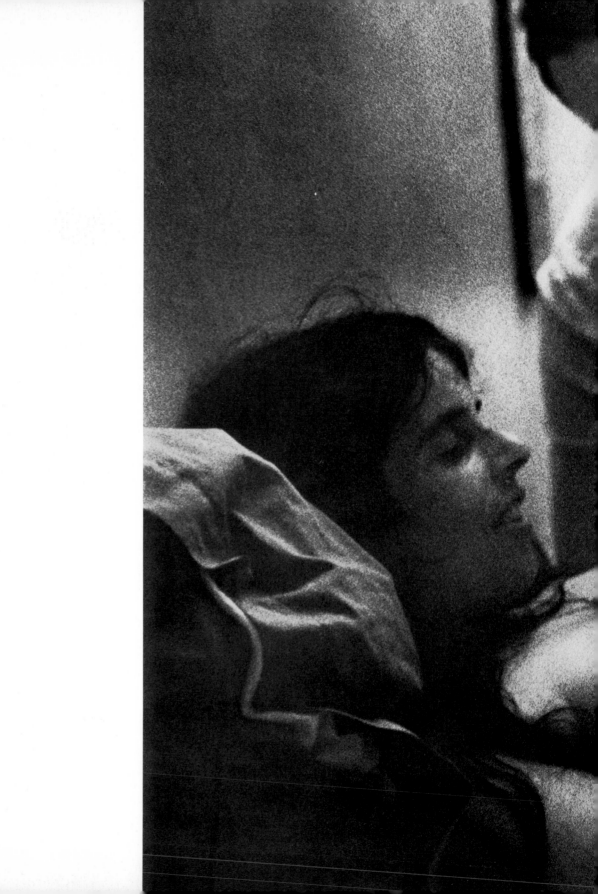

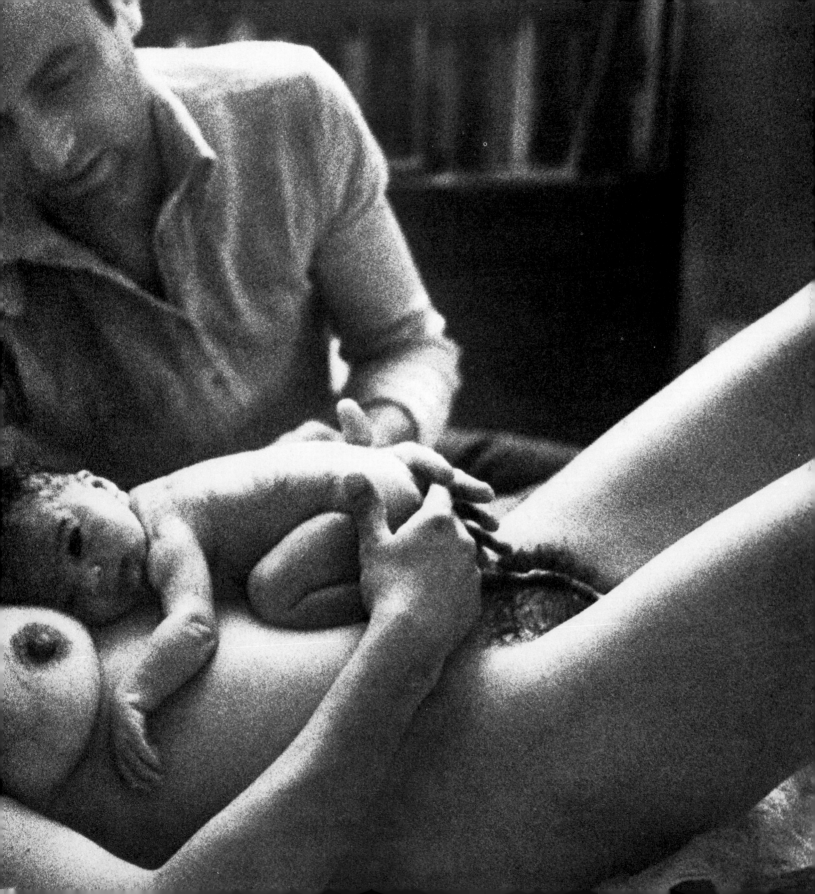

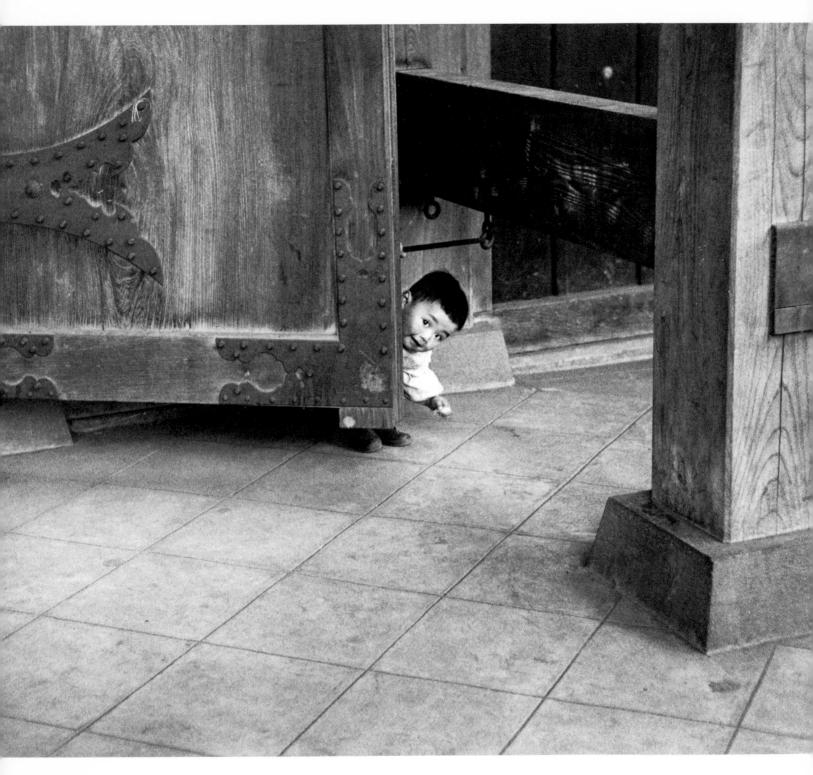

CHARLES RYCROFT

Charles Rycroft has been a psychoanalyst since 1947. He has contributed extensively to literary and professional journals in both Britain and the United States. His books include a study of Wilhelm Reich, called *Reich, Anxiety and Neurosis, Psychoanalysis Observed,* and *Imagination and Reality.*

The psyche and the senses

The sensations arising in our sense-organs are in themselves meaningless physiological phenomena, but are converted into significant psychological experiences by our mind, which does not just passively receive and record sensations but, in addition, also actively selects, transforms and organizes them to construct and create those experiences which comprise our identity and biography. All experience, then, is a creative compound between sensations passively received and imaginative activity which interprets and organizes them.

The most obvious mental quality possessed by human beings is the capacity to be conscious. Human beings, like animals, perceive and act but, unlike animals, we also know that we perceive and act, and at some point in our childhood we acquire the additional capacity to be self-conscious, to know that we know, and to reflect on the sensations we receive, the actions we perform, the experiences we have. As soon as we have acquired self-consciousness, it becomes possible for us to reflect upon the sensations we have and to compare them with other sensations we have previously had; and, furthermore, to anticipate, with either pleasure or dread, the possibility that we may have further sensations and experiences in the future. Consciousness, and, more particularly, self-consciousness, introduces, therefore, an element of critical comparison into all experience, and sensations cease to be isolated, discrete events but become instead experiences which derive their meaning and value from comparison with prior experiences. To an extent which varies with our age, education and sophistication, experiences contain a critical, comparative element which derives from our earlier experiences and from our reflective capacity, not from the sensations themselves. To take a simple example; a child's experience of his first meal at school does not consist simply of the taste of the food he receives. It includes also an evaluation of whether it tastes nicer or nastier than the food he receives at home and the anticipation that later meals at school will resemble it, an anticipation which will fill him with hope or foreboding, depending not only on his comparison of the taste of home and school food but also on whether he has dreaded or looked forward to going to school. What I am suggesting here is that the experience of, for instance, eating food, contains meanings which cannot be attributed to, or deduced from, the sensations of eating it, but which derive from the total psychological context in which the sensations have been perceived.

The same point can usefully be made in another way. Since consciousness is individual, and we each have a continuous sense of our own unique being, which is maintained despite the apparent discontinuities created by sleep, general anaesthetics, concussion etc., all sensational events become experiences in the process of being assimilated into that continuum of being that constitutes our identity. They are construed and interpreted in the light of our previous experiences and after being assimilated and construed they become part of us and influence the meaning we attach to all later experiences.

There are, however, two exceptions to the generalization that all sensations can be converted into experiences by comparison with prior similar sensations. The first is the infant's first contact with the outside world immediately after birth. Although none of us can remember them, we must all have had entirely novel sensations of noise and light, of cold air on our skin, of being handled, immediately after we were born. All the evidence suggests that this sudden bombardment with novel sensations was extremely unpleasant and bewildering, and mothering the new-born seems largely to consist of providing them with conditions which simulate the peace, darkness and warmth of the womb, while at the same time converting them to the belief that sensation can be enjoyable and satisfying. But it remains true throughout life that we view sensation as a mixed blessing; although sensations can be enjoyable, exciting, stimulating, enriching, there are limits to the amount of stimulation we can tolerate, beyond which sensation and consciousness become a burden from which we seek oblivion in sleep.

The second exception is adolescence, when both body and mind acquire new potentialities, erotic, emotional, intellectual and aesthetic. At this time physiological changes produce concomitant changes in both the range and intensity of sensations and in the capacity of the psyche to convert its intake of sensations into significant experiences, these being so great as to constitute a dialectical transformation of the quality of all experience. Although, objectively speaking, pictures will have been seen before, music heard before, people loved and touched before, adolescence is often remembered as a time when pictures and music and love were encountered for the first time and as revelations. The world is perceived and experienced through new eyes, and in two respects adolescence may resemble life immediately after birth when the sensory world was encountered for the first time; it may be bewildering and the need for intermittent relief from sensation in sleep may be enormous.

Our consciousness of our own continuous being compels us, therefore, to convert the physical sensations we receive into mental experiences which derive their significance from the place they occupy in our biography and from the connections we establish between them and all our other experiences. As a result, the meaning any perceptual event has depends less on the sensation itself than on the age, the sex, the education, the occupation, the health, of the perceiver. This is perhaps most obviously true of sensations produced by works of art. Looking at, say,

Botticelli's *Birth of Venus* will be a very different experience for a child, a teenager, a man, a woman, an artist, an art dealer, and an old person who knows he is near to death, even though the painting may produce an identical image on their respective retinas.

The dependence of the meaning of experiences on the psyche of the experiencer can, on occasion, lead to striking discrepancies between sensations and the experience constructed round them. An Australian woman was once walking through Covent Garden when she suddenly burst into tears: the scent of a consignment of eucalyptus blossom in the market had brought back to her vivid overwhelming recollections of the Australian bush, which she had not seen for many years. This transformation of a pleasant, in itself trivial, sensation into a distressing, powerful emotional experience of homesickness was due, I suspect, to a conflict between wishes to forget and to remember, to break with the past and to preserve a feeling of continuity with it. A rather similar conflict must, one surmises, have been present in Proust's mind when he tasted the madeleine which started him on his *A la recherche du temps perdu*. I shall return later to a discussion of the effects on sensation and experience of attempts by the psyche to disown parts of its experience.

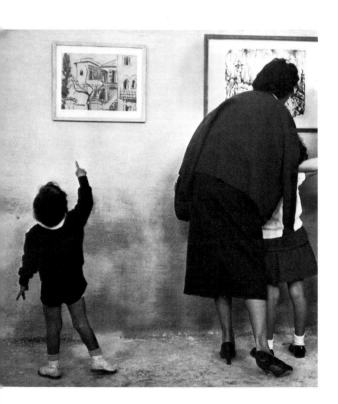

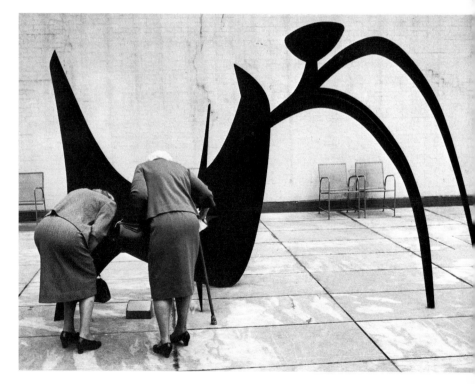

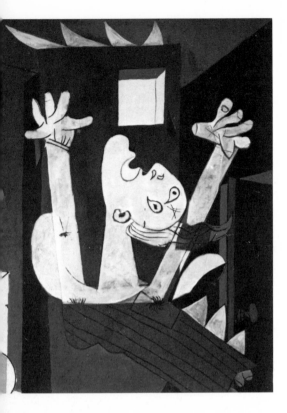

Detail from Picasso's *Guernica*.

It is perhaps enlightening to liken the psyche's conversion of physical sensations into mental experiences to the attitude of an organism towards objects which come close enough to it to be ingested. Some will be ignored as irrelevant, others will be tasted but spat out in disgust, others will be ingested but later expelled as useless and unassimilable. Some, however, will be digested, absorbed and assimilated into the structure of, in one case, the body and, in the other case, the mind, the selection being made on the basis of the physiological and psychological needs of the organism and mind respectively.

This analogy cannot, however, be taken too far, since it is unfortunately not true that we have full freedom of choice in our psychological diet and can always expel disagreeable sensations and events without assimilating them into our psyches. If we had such freedom, unhappy childhoods, deprivations and experiences of maltreatment and cruelty would leave people unharmed. But the analogy does, nonetheless, draw attention to the fact that what we perceive and the interpretation we put on sensations is affected by our psychological needs. If we are hungry, we will be all eyes for food. If we are in love, we will be quick to notice women who resemble the loved one and may momentarily mistake them for her. If we are touched by someone we love, it will be pleasant, perhaps even thrilling, whereas an identical touch by someone we dislike or fear will be distasteful. And occurrences which at one phase of our life are enjoyable and significant may at another mean nothing to us. In general, the meaning given to any sensation depends on the perceiver's mental attitude towards the source of the sensation, and on his expectations from that source.

There exists, however, a type of occurrence in which sensations are forced upon consciousness and the psyche which it has no option but to perceive, but which it is equally unable to assimilate and convert into experiences of a meaningful, let alone enriching, kind. These are the sensations produced by traumatic events, that is by totally unexpected disastrous events, such as earthquakes, car or plane accidents, or sexual and other physical violations. The immediate effect of such experiences is a state of shock, in which the victim is unable to comprehend what has happened to him. He may, if he is lucky, get over it, but he will not have been enriched by it. Memories of traumatic events are more like foreign bodies embedded in the psyche than essential parts of it, since they remain disconnected from the continuum of experience.

In striking contrast to memories of traumatic events, which are conscious but are not true parts of the psyche, are repressed parts of the self, which are unconscious and yet do form parts of the psyche. These are parts of the self, containing memories, wishes and emotions which were once conscious but have been disowned and repressed at some time in the past, usually in childhood, in order to avoid confrontations with figures in the outside world, typically parents who, it is imagined – often rightly – would disapprove of them and withdraw security and affection if they received expression. These repressed parts of the self continue,

72

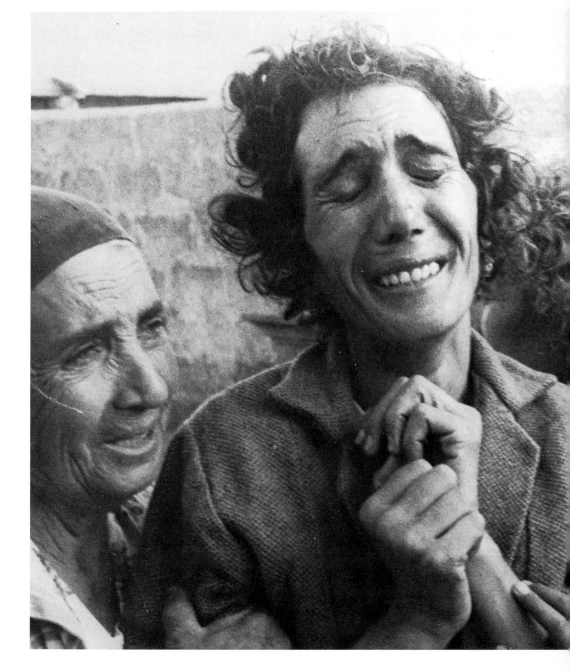

Her husband has just been killed.

René Magritte, *The Rape*, 1945.

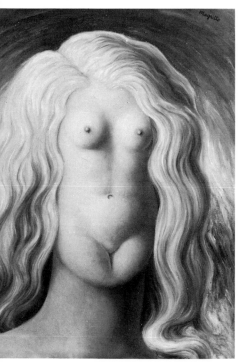

however, to crave expression and as a result the repressing, disowning, central psyche has to avoid becoming conscious of those features of the present which might resonate and revive them. This repression leads inevitably to impoverishment of both sensation and experience.

If, for instance, someone as a child represses his sexual and aggressive potentialities, he will as an adult be an inhibited, meek person with an impaired capacity for enjoying erotic and assertive situations. Or if someone has disowned his childhood *en bloc* and can no longer remember what it was like to be a child, his capacity to enjoy and understand children will be impoverished. Or if someone has disowned all feeling, his capacity to love and to enjoy the arts will be reduced. In all these all-too-common instances, disowning by the psyche of parts of itself and its own past experience reduces the individual's capacity to appreciate sensations and convert them into experiences. It is as though, in the process of converting sensations into significant experiences, the psyche acts as a resonator which adds to all present perceptions harmonics derived from its past, and repression impoverishes experience by cutting out some of the possible harmonics. Or, to shift from a musical to a linguistic metaphor, repression reduces the number of meanings – and the total intensity of meanings – that can be attributed to messages received from the senses.

Another mental quality involved in the conversion of sensations into experiences is the capacity to attach symbolic meanings to them. It is characteristic of human beings, as opposed to animals, that they are capable of accepting symbolic substitutes for the original objects of instinctual wishes, so that, for instance, listening and looking can become substitutes for eating, intellectual curiosity can become a substitute for wishes to explore one's own and other people's bodies, and nature and ideals can be loved as though they were people. Although the connection between mental 'sublimated' activities and biological drives was originally discovered during investigation of the meaning of dreams, neurotic symptoms and inhibitions, it is also revealed by language, which allows one to describe music as the food of love, to describe inquisitive people as 'nosey' and curiosity as devouring, to personify nature as a mother, and to attribute gender to ideals, institutions, countries and even abstract ideas. It would seem indeed that built into the psyche is a symbolic or metaphorical network of connections and resonances which make us react to all the objects we perceive as though they were to a greater or lesser extent representatives, substitutes or equivalents of people, bodies, or parts of bodies, and that this symbolic network is responsible for our imaginative, as opposed to literal, response to what we perceive.

This capacity of the mind to endow all its perceptions with additional symbolic meanings can be exemplified by our responses to scenery and architecture. It is, for instance, what makes us feel that bleak countrysides are unfriendly and unwelcoming but that lush valleys are friendly and welcoming, that mountains, cliffs and large buildings are majestic and awe-inspiring, that tall buildings, particularly if they lack windows, are austere and forbidding, and that houses with bay windows and wings coming out to meet one are inviting. In all these instances we react to things – scenery and buildings – as though they were people who might embrace, ignore or cold-shoulder us. And it is the same symbolizing capacity of the mind which is responsible for what has become known as Freudian symbolism, that is the tendency to endow even inanimate objects with gender on the basis of any discernible resemblance to sexual organs.

Although there is much that remains obscure and controversial about the connections between repression and symbolization, it seems that some measure of repression of instinctual impulses is necessary to initiate the formation of symbols, but that excessive repression diminishes the capacity to endow the sensory world with symbolic meanings. Although it would be rational to be immune to the pathetic fallacy and to perceive scenery as only geological formations, buildings as only bricks and mortar, paintings as only pigments on a canvas, something important is lost if one cannot react to them in terms of the symbolism and metaphor that can be read into them – and that in the case of artefacts such as paintings has in fact been written into them. Repression, therefore, impoverishes appreciation of the sensory world by reducing the symbolic resonances and meanings that can be read into sensations.

It would seem, too, that these symbolic resonances and meanings hark back to infancy, before the discrete objects that compose our sensory world were recognized as entities in themselves but were still regarded as extensions of ourselves or our mothers; and when all pleasurable sensations were interpreted as evidence of her love and all painful ones as evidence of her neglect or hostility.

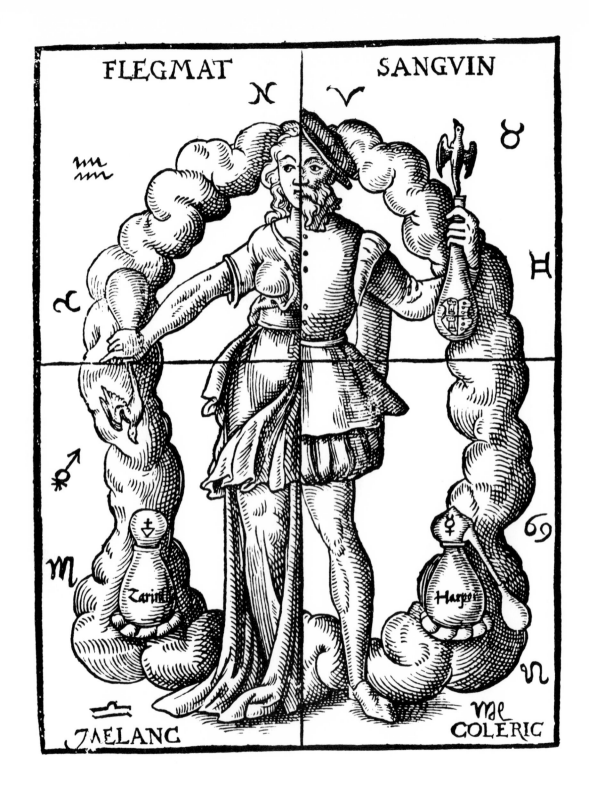

IAN F. BAKER

In this chapter, Ian Baker, a Jungian analyst, looks at the psychological characteristics of artists to discover what it is that gives them the ability to be creative.

The four humours: engraving from W. Thurneysser, *Quinta Essentia*, 1574.

Character and creativity

Depth psychology has attempted to apply itself to most areas of life and living, not least to the way the artist functions. Attempts have been made to account for the psychic causes and reasons why an artist is an artist, be he a writer, painter, musician or whatever. We only have to think of Freud's article on Leonardo da Vinci, where da Vinci's homosexuality is emphasized, or more recent studies such as E. and R. Sterba's work on Beethoven, where it is postulated that the paranoid nature of Beethoven's personal relationships does not, in fact, find expression in his musical creation. There has been a flood of books and articles trying in part to understand, in part to explain away, why the artist creates art.

These numerous studies have caused outbursts of justifiable criticism, snorts of frustration, and snarls of irritation. What does a psychologist know about the way an artist ticks? What does it matter if Leonardo was homosexual? What right does a psychologist have to turn a psychopathological spotlight onto the creative work of an artist or, for that matter, to say that unconscious creative output necessarily reflects the conscious problems of the artist? But the strongest criticism strikes a deeper level. Does not the psychologist, in fact, kill the spontaneous response of the psychologically unarmed reader, listener, viewer? Can we let ourselves float away into the magical world of *The Wind in the Willows* if we are nagged by the thought that its author was writing purely out of his infantile fantasy? Can we listen again to Schumann if we ask all the time if his music was not the expression of his manic-depressive psychosis? Can we look at Paul Klee and not at the same time see his schizophrenia? But behind this is a deeper malaise. We psychologists assert that we seek broader horizons for man's existence, deeper insight into his inner workings, higher goals for his intellect, greater spontaneity in his passions, and more committed concern in the interpersonal and intersocial relationships he must have. The artist expresses the refinements of all these strivings. He reaches out beyond the limit of average experience and extends his world beyond the limits of so-called normal perception. In the eyes of run-of-the-mill psychologists, this means that he is abnormal – not above normal, but abnormal. And abnormal is psychopathological. Thus the artist, somewhere or other, must be sick!

This, however, is not just the fault of psychology. Our education lays far too much stress on criticism. And criticism gets more and more negative. We are subtly being

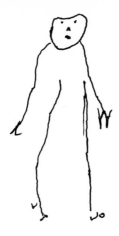

conditioned to find what we do not like, what we do not enjoy, what offends our aesthetic sensibility. Reviews become more and more levelling attacks, and the faint words of appreciation disappear in a swamp of disdain and dislike. Is it surprising then that our world seems to be in decline and that we apologize for our likes and our pleasures, possibly because we no longer dare or care to describe them?

I am supposed to contribute something about what it feels like to create, but I am reluctant for so many reasons, some of which have been touched upon. And behind is this feeling of wanting to throw my pencil across the room. The words come to mind of an analytical psychologist who did his best to instil some common sense into my training. He said, in passing, 'When you get a creative artist, a real artist, in your practice, watch it that you never touch the artistic spot in him. If you do, you will squash him as an artist.' I had visions of wearing special protective gloves when my treatment of this neurotic or psychotic patient got close to his artistic core. But how would I recognize it, not being an artist myself? What is this odd thing which makes an artist special? And what if the artist had not as yet proved himself by bringing out some big work reviewed in the right magazine and is still only a latent artist? And for that matter, isn't everyone somewhere or other at even a minimal level a small artist, even if all he ever managed to create is some small pot at a night school? The artist, after all, is not just the major name on the artistic horizon – the composer whose works are immediately performed at the next large festival, the painter whose paintings are promptly bought as they leave the studio, the poet whose next volume is eagerly awaited by public and critic alike. The term must cover anyone who tries to create something of himself and from himself. In fact, anyone concerned with heightening his perceptions or broadening the spectrum of sense – even if not externally productive – is certainly internally creative.

In a way I think that my training analyst was right. In another way, he was wrong. For though you could easily distort the flow of creative energy within an artistic person, even so, at the same time you sense that the artistic spark is not something which is so easily extinguished. So maybe creative man is safe from psychologists – at least until he's dead and then becomes a target for posthumous assassination.

For that matter, what harm can be done to the artist's creative output if it is established that creativity, neurosis, and psychosis can exist side by side? The dilemma seems to be as follows. Art has its place in the depths of the human psyche. Art is produced by creative man. The psyche is understood, to a small degree at least, by the psychologist. But on the one hand, we have the inability of the true artist to explain what occurs to him when he is seized within the creative process. On the other hand, we have the psychologist who is not an artist trying to superimpose patterns of understanding upon something which he can never understand.

The ideal would be to find the artist-psychologist who could explain to us both sides of the coin. But does such a person exist? And would he, in any event, be able to describe clearly the two sides of his being? Even if such a paragon existed, would

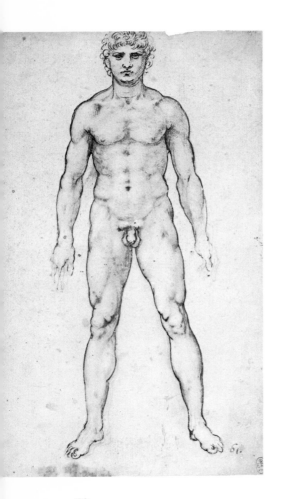

the artist in him in the one ivory tower be able to speak to the psychologist in him in another ivory tower? It would seem to be well nigh impossible because he would have, in fact, to describe how he feels when he initially notices the artistic spark within him. He would then have to describe the transformation of that spark into some, perhaps indescribable, form of energy which reaches out within his being towards expression and finally to describe the conscious attitude to the final product, that is, the work of art. He would be asked to listen to two voices; the one being the voice speaking to us directly through the work of art, the other the voice *of the artist* communicating *through* his work of art. But then we are left with the link unexplained between the end product and the process of creation. For the psychologist this is difficult. Psychologists have as much right as anyone to try to investigate complex psychic processes. But any psychologist who is honest enough to submit to his own and his patient's experiences must also admit to being in the dark when it comes to explaining rationally such basic problems as creation and life. Until a true dialogue can take place in all openness between an artist and a psychologist upon this very point, then we will have to accept our inability to perceive even remotely just what it all feels like.

We could perhaps put it this way: true art is always totally new and totally old. It seems to come from the deepest layers of mankind's experience. It comes through to us between the lines of poetry, between the strains of music, between the colours of painting. It causes an individual moment of recognition. It arouses immediate emotion. It strikes us with its clarity and beauty. But we are left incapable of describing what it is, even though we know that we recognize it. It comes from some deep layer within us which we feel that we cannot define, and it is beyond the confines of sanity and insanity, of normality and abnormality.

We have before us, then, the expression of something unconscious. But there is more to it than that, for a work of art, objectively, is totally independent. Not only that, it is totally independent of the artist as individual. The composer, having written his music, must let that music be heard. The painter, having painted his picture, must let it be observed. The poet, having written his poem, must let it be spoken.

We must now turn to the theory, often raised, that typology, as it is called, helps us to understand the artist. But what do we mean by typology? We might start by saying that man has always attempted to find not his similarities but his dissimilarities; that, in order to understand the diversity of his nature, he has tried to see himself in terms of types. If we go back as far as Hippocrates, we find him dividing the body into the four elements of earth, air, water, and fire. These four elements were, in Hippocrates' theory, linked in some way to substances to be found in the body, such as blood, phlegm, bile and urine. Hippocrates was followed some centuries later by Galen who talked of the four humours: the sanguine, the choleric, the melancholic, and the phlegmatic. These four subdivisions seemed to satisfy man's need for an explanation of his uniqueness up until some hundred years ago when, with the development of medical science and of psychology, people became less content to understand, sympathize with, or dislike each other because of 'humours'. New attempts at research were made to find new means of delineating human differences both physical and psychic. And perhaps the most important of these researchers was Kretschmer. What Kretschmer attempted was to establish a link between physique and character. His thesis was that certain bodily types link with certain forms of insanity; not only that, but that this link can also be found in people who are normal and sane. But Kretschmer opened also the floodgates for further theories and for further subdivisions; the result was frightful confusion. Reading these later works, one is left with the impression that the best description by far was made in terms of 'humours', for at least that is understandable. One turns then with some relief to Jung's publication of 1921, entitled *Psychological Types*. In this work, Jung places man in his historical context and attempts to describe him in terms of attitude and of function. He claims that two attitudes – extraversion and introversion – are discernible in man, and that furthermore these attitudes are linked to one or more of four basic psychological functions: sensation, intuition, feeling, and thinking.

But what does Jung mean by extraversion and introversion? We must, in the first place, guard ourselves against confusion of Jung's interpretation of the meaning of these two attitudes and the general understanding of extraversion and introversion as being something on the lines of, on the one hand, superficiality and, on the other, morbid retirement from active life. For Jung means far more than seeing the extravert as the person who makes the party go, and the introvert as the person who prefers to stay at home in the evening.

What Jung implies is that there are two distinct ways in which people approach objects around them. It is simpler to understand what Jung meant if one returns to his own original description: 'Quite generally, one could describe the introverted standpoint as one that under all circumstances sets the self and the subjective psychological processes above the object and the objective process, or at any rate, holds its ground against the object – the extraverted standpoint, on the other hand, sets the subject below the object, whereby the object receives the predominant value. The subject always has secondary importance; the subjective process appears at times merely as a disturbing or superfluous accessory to objective events.' It is very important to remember that though we appear to have one of these attitudes as dominant, the other attitude is always present even if in diminished form. Therefore, you cannot have someone who is totally extraverted or someone who is totally introverted. Furthermore, both attitudes are, of course, valid even though difficulties of understanding must arise when an extreme extravert meets an extreme introvert. The extravert, who orients himself by habit through the world outside himself, will naturally find it difficult to reach a common line of communication with someone for whom the object is but a secondary and indirect factor in his life.

The habitual attitude, be it extraversion or introversion, can also cause difficulties, particularly if the person finds himself in a society in which his opposite attitude is more closely associated to the collective norms of behaviour. Furthermore, any attempt to overadapt to the opposite attitude, for whatever reason, can only lead to psychic damage: not only, for example, will the introvert who plays at being extraverted appear ill-adapted, he will also be violating his natural manner of perceiving life. It does not need any great stretch of the imagination to conceive of such cases – only think what would go wrong if two extraverted parents with an introverted child attempted to condition the child to react to the world according to *their* attitude.

Valuable though this may be, it is not sufficient, of course, to divide people up simply into extraverted and introverted groups. Jung makes a further subdivision in terms of what he calls the four functions: thinking, feeling, intuition, and sensation. But what does Jung really mean by a psychic function? He describes it as 'a certain form of psychic activity that remains theoretically the same under varying circumstances'. The thinking function implies the apprehension of what is around and in us through thought and cognition. Data are collected, and used logically. Thinking, then, is a rational function. The other rational function, in Jung's terms, is feeling. Feeling as a function is, for Jung, a matter of evaluation and judgment more than pure emotion. This evaluation or judgment is subject to a 'feeling' of something being attractive or unattractive, acceptable or not acceptable. Feeling evaluates or devaluates. The distinction between feeling and general emotion is that the feeling type can *explain* why he reacts in one way or another to the object. Sensation and intuition are the irrational functions in that they are concerned more with perception than with judgment and more with sensing than with evaluating. Sensation registers all sensory data around us, but its limits are in the fact that it *merely* registers what is around us or what qualities this person or object has. Intuition is also a function of perception but is more difficult to describe because it uses not so much the conscious senses as unconscious perceptions. Intuition, then, registers not so much the actual but the inherent quality of the object. A basic example of the difference is that the sensation function takes in all the details of a room while intuition, paying little regard to detail, will pick up the atmosphere and the unconscious implications of what is going on in that room.

We have, then, the two rational functions and two irrational functions. But each of these two groups is mutually exclusive. You cannot have thinking *and* feeling; you cannot have sensation *and* intuition. And though we have all four functions within us, we have, as it were, a natural bent for one of them. We could say that we have 'naturally' a main function, be it thinking, feeling, intuition, or sensation. But, as we have seen from the description of the workings of these functions, one function is not sufficient to allow man to make his way through life adequately. Observation indicates that we have a main function, but this main function is inadequate on its own. It needs to be coloured by an auxiliary function. If we take, for example, a thinking type, we will see that his thinking will be of little use to him unless he can

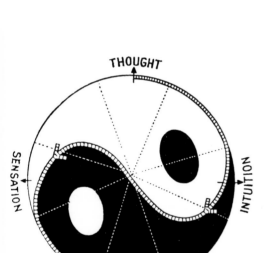

C. G. Jung's 'Compass of the psyche'.

81

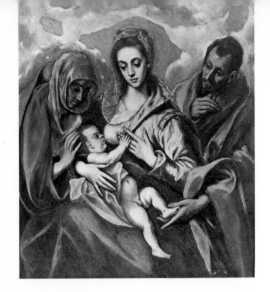

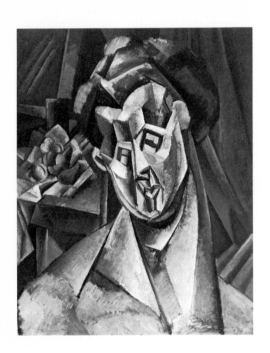

El Greco, *Virgin of the Good Milk*, 1590–98.

Picasso, *Woman with Pears*, 1909.

colour it with sensation, turning the pure thinking into the direction of empirical thinking; or he may need intuition, which will lead his thinking more into speculative areas. The more man develops, the more he finds he is able to use a third function. But it would seem impossible for all four functions to be available to one and the same person. One function always remains inferior, or at least not readily available. Thus, a thinking type will suffer from the lack of feeling, and the feeling type will suffer equally from the lack of the thinking function. Or, in other words, the inferior function remains unconscious – which does not, however, mean that the inferior function is not there. For the inferior function has a peculiar quality in that, because of its lack of availability to consciousness, it intrudes into life in an inadequate way. It has also a peculiar fascination, and it can be very often found that life partners, say married couples, may well have the opposite functions. If recognized, this can provide positive, constructive compensation; if unrecognized, perpetual quarrel and misunderstanding.

It sounds, from what has gone before, as if we have four types of people. But, in fact, there are eight types, in that each function can be either extraverted or introverted. And it must be briefly pointed out that in that rare thing, a normal development, a human being lives according to his natural attitude be it extraverted or introverted, develops a main function and, as life progresses, develops also an auxiliary and a third function, and recognizes the values of what must always be the inferior function. Conversely, one must recognize the limping development of a person who has the wrong attitude thrust upon him and is conditioned to live in terms of the wrong function.

Can this theory be used in any way to facilitate the difficulties we experience in our attempts to understand the manifold facets of the artist's psychic life? Can we be as bold as Herbert Read and say that Picasso in his cubist period was working 'purely intuitively'? Or that El Greco is an artist who clearly belongs to the introverted sensation type? Can we blindly accept from the created work of Rubens that Rubens was himself an extraverted sensation type or that Piero della Francesca was an extraverted intuitive? Or, turning to composers, can we agree that 'Music can, of course, express the other function types, but it finds its normal and its most profound development in the expression of the introverted intuitive mode of consciousness'? This can only be guesswork. The proof of the validity of such assessments could only be established by testing a known contemporary artist for his typology and then viewing his finished works to see if this assessment fits with the type given to him. We most probably would find that the conscious function of our artist has little to do with the function and attitude inherent in his painting. We would also probably find that there would be widely different views on the typology exhibited through the created work of art. And we would be left with a number of questions such as what we mean by extraverted or introverted art. Are the Haydn Masses more extravert than the Bach B minor? Is Francis Bacon more introverted in his painting than Henry Moore in his sculpture?

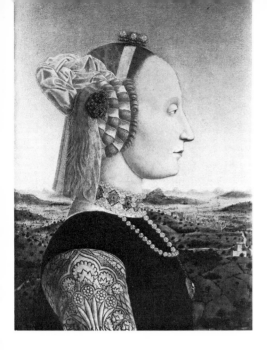

Piero della Francesca, *Duchess of Urbino*, c.1472.

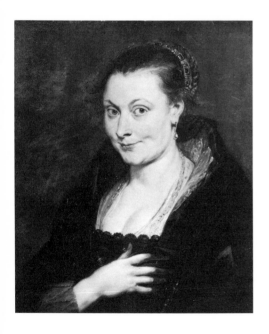

Rubens, *Portrait of Isabella Brant*, c.1620.

We seem to be getting ourselves caught in a trap inherent in many a psychological theory; namely, of making the theory fit the case and thus eliminating the possibility of approaching each 'case' as a unique entity. It also implies a basic misunderstanding of typology as such, and we should remind ourselves of the following points.

From a practical day-to-day viewpoint, an understanding of our individual typology can assist us in understanding how we function in the outer world, how we relate to our fellow men and, what is more important, where our difficulties lie in adaptation to the outer world. But the more we understand our functioning and the more we attune to our attitude, the more we realize how flexible we must be. We naturally function best through our main function and through our habitual attitude, but we find that, with the diversity of human encounters, we must, as it were, fluctuate between functions and tone down our dominant attitude. But this is not always possible. In moments of stress and in times of conflict we seem naturally to retreat into a rigid stance based upon dominant attitude and main function.

The inherent danger in such a theory is that the theory becomes its own answer. You either fit into one of the type categories or you are an outsider and an oddball. But this can never be the case, and once we try to establish a rigid code of types we defeat our own purpose which is, after all, to broaden rather than limit the scope of our functioning. For the expression of the type is coloured by many other factors, such as personality structure, temperament, background and all that makes the individual what he is. We are first and foremost individuals and only secondarily people who somewhere seem to lean towards one of the eight types.

A question strikes us when we talk of the creative artist. Does he function best as artist when he uses his main function, or does he in fact become creative when there is either a slight switch from balance between functions, or does he become creative when he is caught by his inferior function? If we remember that the inferior function is in the unconscious, and that it seems that the root of artistic expression is to be found in the deeper layers of the unconscious, would it not then be likely that the creative spark is activated and fuelled by that inferior function? Now this is going against what has already been written about typology and art. Sir Herbert Read has attempted an understanding of the psychological implications of temperament and feeling in the artist and has used the Jungian approach to typology. But he seems to take as his premise that the artist, in order to create, must work through his main function. I have already mentioned his views on El Greco and Picasso and composers in general.

But this viewpoint seems to imply that the artist works through his conscious function; it further seems to imply a certain awareness on the part of the artist which is not necessarily the case. It does not seem to be true or capable of any proof that the artist functions on a conscious level when he is at work. On the contrary, many artists will describe their feelings when being creative as being diffuse, even painful, and certainly not smoothly comfortable. It is as if they describe an urge which they

83

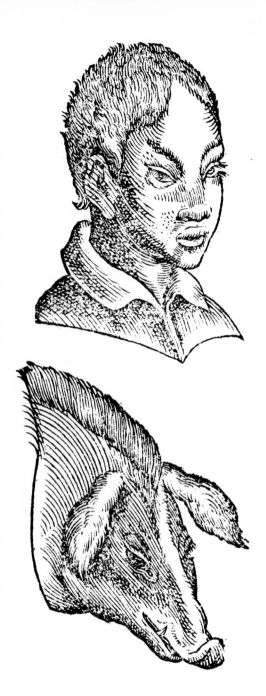

cannot account for and a drive, in the general sense of the term, which cannot be suppressed. We might describe this as a yearning or an itch. But however we describe it, it certainly sounds like a vacuum or void which must at all cost be filled. This vacuum or void causes restless tension which must be appeased. If you are near an artist who is caught by this tension, you may dismiss his mood as something to do with his being caught up in his 'artistic temperament'. But what is this so-called and much-laboured term 'artistic temperament'? To the outsider it appears unrelated, objectless, volatile and dramatic. It may also appear childlike, moody and affected, even inflated. It is used as an excuse for all sorts of inadequate expressions of behaviour, but at the same time it calls for you to leave the person alone until he sorts it out.

To the outsider, the artist at this moment may appear disjointed, distracted, or 'spaced out'. He appears caught by something beyond his control and yet which he must contain until it takes form. He is 'not himself'. To the observer he may appear pained and cramped, or he may have that tranquil aloofness which we often see in the faces of women in the last month of pregnancy. There is both suspension and tension but, be it a child or a poem, something has got to come out. And it seems inevitable that the birth must be accompanied by suffering.

With the artist, we could say that this suffering is necessary. But suffering is caused by a dilemma, by a conflict, by the inevitability of solution to an inner conflict. And it is accompanied by self-doubt and insecurity, together with a certain knowledge that this mood will not pass until something has been 'formed' and that conception, gestation and creation are part and parcel of one and the same scheme.

In this, it would appear that the total psyche is involved. It is not just the ego in collusion with the main function, but consciousness and unconsciousness at work together. When the total psyche is involved, we have as little control over it as we would have over our dreams. We cannot just call into use our better parts and we cannot plaster over our inferior being.

Now we have come into a peculiar area. We all must, at various moments in our lives and for a variety of reasons, suppress or ignore or reject or repress parts of our nature, and even our own conscience may not allow us to be our 'real selves'. We cannot just let everything 'hang out', however much we may want to. (And this applies not just to sexuality, even though psychology seems to be morbidly intrigued by that one side of our being.) All schools of psychology explain this element of rejection in a wide variety of terms; Jung described it as the shadow, by which he meant all that a person must, for whatever reason, put aside, away or below. But the shadow is neither totally bad nor totally inferior. It contains what is incompatible with the ego. It will contain what we do not like consciously about our nature, but it may well contain something which we very much need. We may, for example, suppress our ambition because we cannot accept the idea of 'trampling over corpses' to get ahead. But in suppressing natural ambition, we may also suppress a healthy desire to better ourselves.

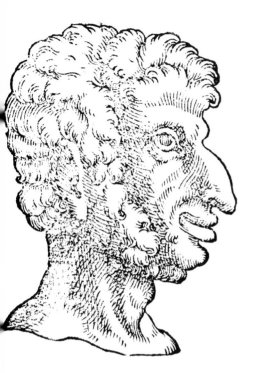

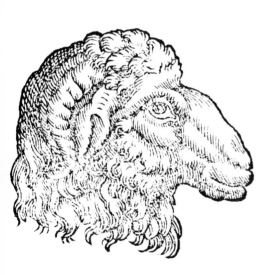

Two illustrations from Giovanni Battista della Porta, *De Humana Physiognomia . . .*, 1593. It suggests close human–animal correspondences for people with certain characteristics.

We usually see our shadow by the process of projection, in that we see it unconsciously, say, in people whom we inexplicably dislike. But the shadow, being unconscious or only partly conscious, also seems to be connected with our inferiority and with our inferior function.

If we think about our own shadow, about what is inferior in us, be it our less respectable sides or our 'animal natures', we may notice not only that we avoid it like the plague, but that it has its own peculiar quality. It seems to want to get at us and to be heard. And when we are not completely in control, it pops up and catches us off guard when we 'aren't ourselves'. It also seems to cry out for expression when no one is there to criticize us for just 'being what we are'.

When we experience this inferior side of our being, we not only feel that we have lost control over what we would 'like' to be, but are ill at ease. In loftier terms we could say we feel we are no longer centred, or that our ego no longer occupies a dominant position in our consciousness. We all have an idea of how best we function at varying levels of existence; we also know the feeling of being 'out of sorts' or 'not with it'. And we might explain these moments by saying that we are not reacting through our main function or our habitual attitude. We might also say we are behaving badly. However we describe it, we know that we are experiencing an uncomfortable state when parts of our nature come up, over which we do not have total control.

If we are careful, though, we may notice that it is just at these moments that we experience other sides of our being which are new to us. We ordinary mortals do all we can to get back on an even keel. The artist, and the generally creative person, however, seems to have a different reaction. It is just in these moments that he feels he must express something in a new dimension. The conflict and the tension shake his balance, and in the no-man's-land between the poles of conflict and tension something new and unconscious may struggle for shape and form. And he lets it happen, without, as in the case of the so-called normal person, trying to pull himself back into shape. It is as if a gap grows within him and through this gap comes purely unconscious material which must be given form. To resist is impossible, because the force of the urge is too strong. And putting off the evil day through mundane activity will not work either, for the more the repression of the creative urge, the stronger it becomes.

The artist must submit to a form of possession which will only subside once the force has been given form. The tension, if abused, leads to neurotic, inadequate behaviour on an external level. But the harnessing of the tension seems to lead to a creative release of the inner conflict. It is not something which just happens, however. It requires, from the artist, first the recognition of the potential value of the tension and then the more difficult direction of the will in order to give it form. It also requires an ability to allow a kind of floating between the typological functioning in order to find which area will best give expression to that which is forcing its way up from the unconscious. This *may* be through the use of the main function; it could equally well be through the use of the less-developed functions or through the opposite to the habitual attitude.

There is another facet to this tension which is hard to describe. The artist must fuse an unconscious force into a conscious mode, be it painting, poetry, music or what have you. It appears to us like integrating something which is as yet disintegrated, or, more generally expressed, putting the bits together or restoring some order to disorder. The artist experiences, as far as we can see, not only a heightened sense of tension, but also a heightened sense of the power to symbolize. It is the opening to symbolic expression which brings the relief. What is this strange process which we call symbolization? Everyone has it, but it seems it is only free to work when the conscious level is lowered, say in moments of distraction, in daydreaming or in sleep when our dreams play with our inner symbols. For the artist, though, there is another possibility in the waking state when symbolization can take place and the symbols of dreams take on concrete and tangible form. The waking ego then copes with the unconscious fantasies and gives them recognizable shape and a new reality. The internal is then made external in an enhanced form. Whether the end result is beautiful or gives rise to response in the beholder, listener or reader seems to be of less importance.

SOCIAL CONDITIONING:
understanding cultural values

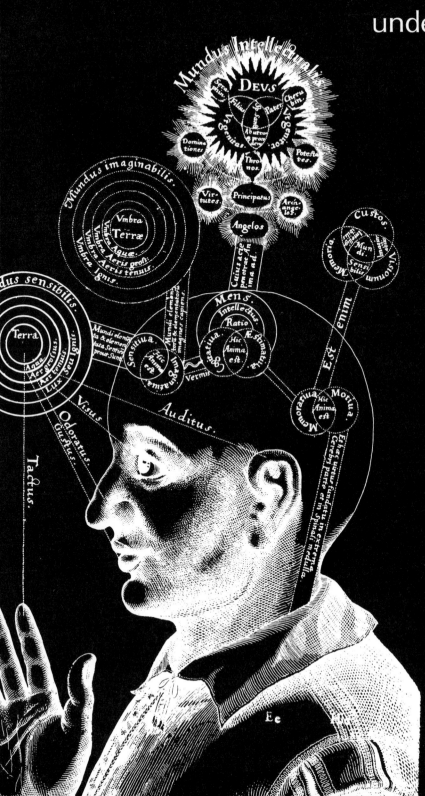

The forming of the five senses is a labour of the entire history of the world down to the present.

Karl Marx

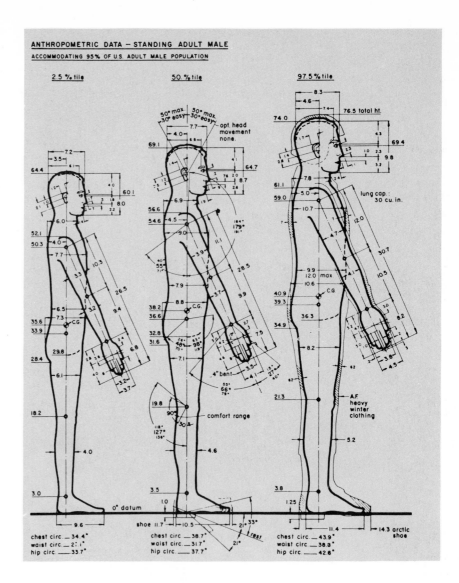

The body is a highly restricted medium of expression. The form it adopts in movement and response expresses social pressure in manifold ways. The care that is given to it, in grooming, feeding and therapy; the theories about what it needs in the way of sleep and exercise, about the stages it should go through, the pains it can stand, its span of life, all the cultural categories in which it is perceived, must correlate closely with the categories in which society is seen insofar as these also draw upon the same culturally processed idea of the body.
Mary Douglas

Lā ilāha illa' Llah
There is no god but God

Muḥammad rasula' Llah
Muḥammad is the Prophet of God

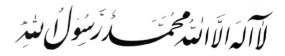

88

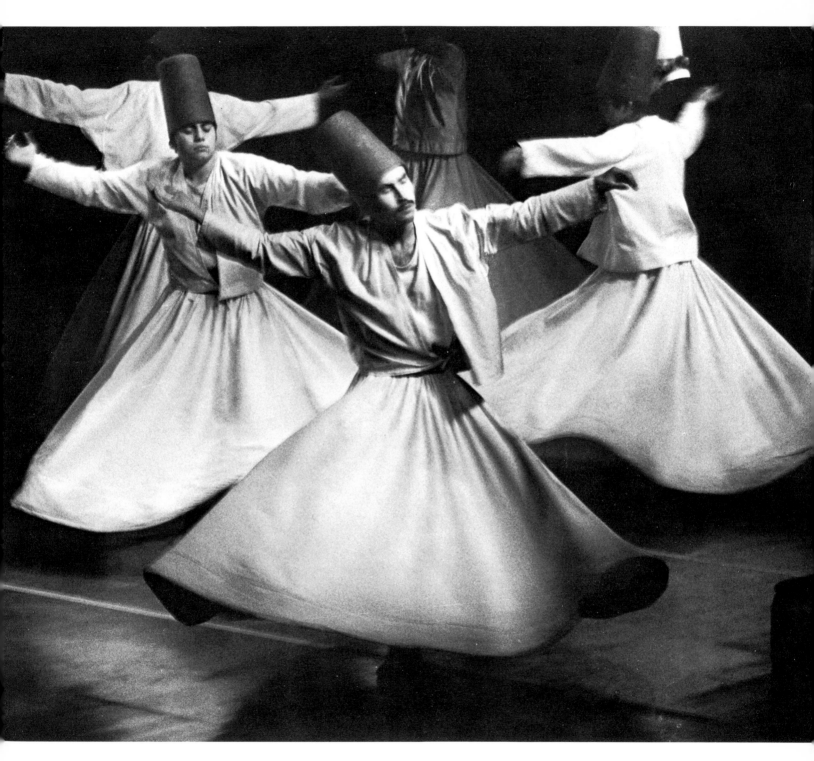

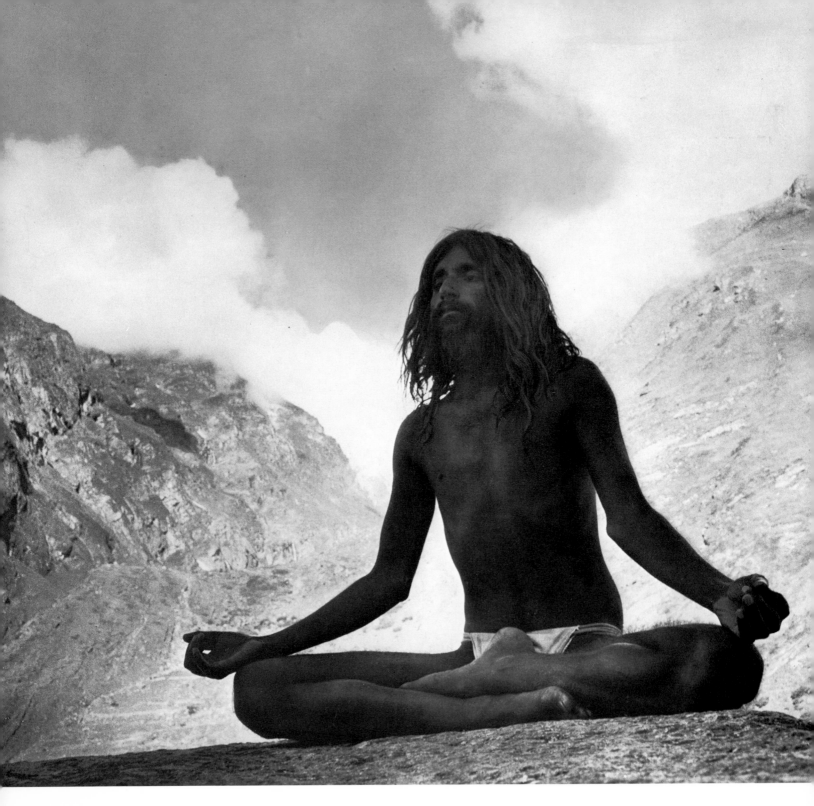

EDMUND LEACH

Of ecstasy and rationality

Sir Edmund Leach is author of *Rethinking Anthropology, A Runaway World, Genius as Myth,* and *Lévi-Strauss.* At the time of writing this chapter he was Professor of Social Anthropology and Provost of King's College, Cambridge. He emphasizes some of the very different attitudes to the senses that have been created by the Western tradition of rationality and compares them with some of the more ecstatic traditions of the East.

The Holy Man of Badrinath.

My main point here is that, as compared with less puritanical traditions, both literate and pre-literate, our Western industrial world is not only more 'rational', in that work tasks are fragmented and the fragments allocated to specialists, but that our tendency to analyse experience into separate sensual aspects — visual, auditory, tactile, etc. — has had the consequence that our total experience is greatly impoverished. Furthermore because such analysis gives the illusion that experience is objective — that a work of art is something other than the total activity of its creator — the relationship between the individual and his or her experience becomes that of critic rather than participant.

The precise relationship between Calvinistic attitudes towards sensual experience and capitalist attitudes towards work and property is a matter of persisting sociological controversy, but, unquestionably, we who live in the West with its heritage of Christian asceticism have become distrustful of our sensual experience. The young Marx considered that the most disastrous aspect of the growth of capitalist industry lay in the alienation of the craftsman from the product of his labour. Wage-labour converted works of art, the expressions of their makers' sensuality, into market commodities in which the individual workman had no interest whatsoever. My present argument is similar: the process of analysis and criticism which leads the contributors to this volume, including myself, to comment on the nature of sensual experience is part of the intellectual game by which, over the past two centuries, the intellectuals and academics of the West have tried to convert the subject-matter of the humanities into a set of experimental psychological and social *sciences.* The cult of the fact has converted subject into object; it has alienated the individual from his feelings.

On the radio and the gramophone, in museums and art galleries, in thousands of programmes on TV and in the cinema, the contemporary educated man has access to the past creations of human sensuality to a degree that has never so far been even remotely possible. But the access is that of observer, not of participant-creator. In the countries of the Christian tradition a higher proportion of the population is literate and (in a bookish sense) 'educated' than ever before, yet there can have been few past civilizations in which, comparatively speaking, so few adults have ever indulged themselves in total emotional exultation or in which experience of this kind was viewed with such deep suspicion.

The sixteenth-century Puritans burnt their ecstatic illiterate neighbours as witches, and a corresponding Establishment hatred of the permissive society still prevails. But sixteenth-century Puritans were only a zealous minority in a world where the majority shared the secular libertarian values of Vanity Fair. Today things are the other way round. Insofar as there is really a current vogue of 'permissiveness' (which as an anthropologist I find difficult to detect), it is only a small-scale loosening up by a tiny uninfluential minority in a society which has been dominated by strongly puritanical assumptions for well over 150 years.

Analysis and Synthesis

> And out of the ground the Lord God formed every beast of the field and every fowl of the air; and brought them unto Adam to see what he would call them and whatsoever Adam called every living creature, that was the name thereof (Genesis 2:19).

... but the end of that story was that Adam's curiosity got the better of him, and he found himself separated from God and Paradise and the beasts of the field and the fowls of the air.

A capacity for attaching classifying names to things and creatures and sensations or whatever is a unique peculiarity of human kind. It is a creative act. Things, including the individual senses, become what we perceive them to be because, in giving something a name, we isolate that named thing from its context. Paradoxically, therefore, human language is both constructive and destructive: constructive because it makes the world what it is; destructive because, before things can be pieced together, they must first be torn apart. There is a sin in creativity. Adam's first sin was to taste the fruit of the tree that teaches classification, the tree of the knowledge of good and evil. Too late he realized that, since this tree was paired with the tree of life, its other name was the tree of death.

Human beings have two kinds of knowledge: the knowledge of experience, the residue of past 'feelings', and the knowledge that comes from intellectual understanding. The world is a continuum; so also is experience. If I sit on a pin, my pain, my yelp, my jump, the biochemical reaction of my wounded body, are a single event; the elements of that event only become separable as concepts through the analytical use of language. But in order to have an intellectual understanding of the separated concepts we have to put them back into their original context, we have to engage in synthesis. Analysis and synthesis are interdependent; the first is only a meaningful exercise if it is a preliminary to the second. But all too often we persuade ourselves that analysis is an end in itself.

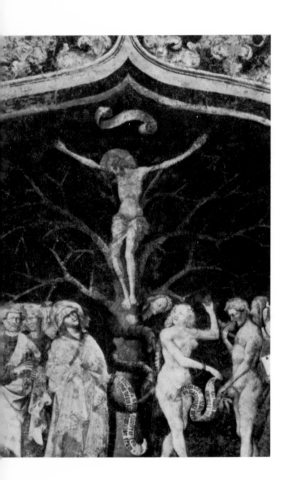

The Tree of Life and Death: wall painting by Giovanni da Modena, c.1420, in the church of San Petronio, Bologna.

92

Paradigms and Syntagms: metaphor and metonymy

There is another important aspect of language which, though quite obvious, is very easy to overlook. All utterances are linear in form and take up time. The event – my sitting on the pin – occupies no time; my description of the event, however reduced, will, at the very least, occupy several seconds or several lines of type. This point is crucial to my whole argument so I must introduce a jargon. In rational analysis, when the various aspects of a single experience are described (pain, yelp, jump, biochemical reaction etc.), the separated facets together form a *syntagm*, a sequential chain – one thing after another, like the words of a sentence. The various facets of the syntagmatic chain are linked together by *metonymy*, in that any one of them can be treated as part for whole, as 'A stands for Apple'. But in actual sensory experience everything happens at once; the different facets are piled one on top of another as in *metaphor*; the yelp 'symbolizes' the pain and *vice versa*. To use jargon again, the yelp is a *paradigm* (a patterned model) of the pain. Notice, however, that whereas the pain is private to my own senses the yelp is public; it is manifest to other people's senses as well as my own.

The major differences between paradigmatic associations (metaphors) on the one hand and syntagmatic chains on the other is that each paradigm represents the whole of whatever is being represented. We can transform one paradigm into another (switch metaphors) but each is complete in itself. If you pile one metaphor on top of another you may convey a richer sense of what is going on but you are not really adding additional information. But a syntagmatic chain is composed of separate component parts, like the letters forming a word or the words forming a sentence; the whole does not exist until you have added all the parts together, though, as in the 'A stands for Apple' case, you can always use metonymy to make a single part stand for an incompleted whole.

The mental operation which we describe as 'thinking' entails repetitive transformations between these two poles. We use analysis to convert paradigmatic (metaphoric) piles of total mental representations into sequentially linked syntagmatic chains of separated items and then prevent the bits from falling apart by resorting to metonymy; or else we operate the other way round, converting syntagmatic chains of separate but linked ideas into unitary paradigms by means of synthesis, using metaphor rather than metonymy to hold things together in the mind.

The consequences of dualistic thinking

Running through all the contributions to this book is the suggestion that, because of our exaggerated admiration for post-Newtonian natural science (which assumes that all 'events' are accessible to objective measurement and are causally related to one another by mechanical links (i.e. by metonymy), we have come to value analysis at the expense of synthesis, and that in the course of this analytical dissection of experience, 'feeling' somehow gets left out. We can measure the pin, the yelp, the jump and the biochemical reaction, but the pain is only a subjective inference.

In over-reaction against this kind of empiricism some protagonists of the counter-culture seem to have been arguing that we ought to pursue an all-embracing synthesized total 'experience' for its own sake without regard for any analysis at all; hypernormal subjective 'feeling' is seen as good in itself.

This is hardly a new idea: it started out with Adam in the Garden of Eden. It has become a problem only because this world and the other world are no longer one and the same. But it is our human capacity for analysis, for separating one thing from another, which has created this distinction.

Anthropologists do not know anything for certain about the origin of religious ideas, but observation of other animals suggests that man is the only creature that is aware that he is destined to die. Moreover, all men know this. All natural languages polarize the concepts 'living' and 'dead'. The living is that which is not yet dead; the dead is that which is no longer alive. The relation between the two is sequential, syntagmatic, and from that it follows that there must be a third category, 'that which the living body has but the dead corpse has not'.

In the course of human history this third factor has been conceptualized in a great variety of ways. Anthropologists and others who have tried to translate the relevant verbal categories into English have used such terms as 'breath', 'life', *psyche*, 'soul', 'spirit', 'ghost', 'power', 'mind', 'potency', 'divine essence'. The common element in these ideas is their *otherness*. The third factor is *not* physical but metaphysical, *not* natural but supernatural.

The creative imagination by which Adam named the animals stemmed from his consciousness of being alone. The total process by which we habitually segment and classify the things in the external world and recognize them as belonging to species entities originates in an introspective self-awareness that 'I' can be distinguished from 'my body'. This Cartesian illusion is directly linked with the universal belief that 'we' ('people like us') can be distinguished from 'they' ('people who are approximately like us in their outward appearance but not like us in their inner essence'). Thus the central persisting human problem is not just 'Who am I?' but 'Who are we?' We, of course, are men. But in what sense are we men? Where and of what kind is the borderline discrimination between man and non-man? God is a human invention devised to answer that question.

The elaboration of the dichotomies 'I' versus 'my body', 'I' versus 'other', 'we' versus 'they' is not restricted to mundane reality; it expands into a whole hierarchy of discriminations, 'friends' versus 'foes', 'recognized neighbours' versus 'unrecognized strangers', 'men' versus 'animals', 'real animals' versus 'monsters', 'gods' versus 'men'. The overall effect is to put man at the centre of the cosmos. 'We' are whatever 'they' are not. But just as we are above the animals, so also we are below the gods. So God is that greater supernatural other, created by man's imagination, which is the locus of life, spirit, power. Notice that we started by discriminating living from dead; we end by discriminating man from God – it is only mortality that separates the two.

In all the religions that are known to ethnography and to history the problem of mortality is central. The basic ideologies are few in number. In the simplest case the cosmos is constructed by inverting our normal experience. Since this world, which is natural, is inhabited by impotent mortal men, the other world, which is supernatural, must be inhabited by omnipotent immortal gods. Religious ritual then serves to establish a bridge between this world and the other world over which potency can flow for the benefit of mortal men. The postulate that when men die their 'spirit', 'life', 'potency' or whatever becomes detached from the mortal carcase but survives in some other mode of existence fits easily into this framework. Just where the souls of deceased ancestors survive is a matter for eschatological argument, but they merge easily with divine powers.

This imaginative intellectual process, whereby everything that is complicated and incomprehensible is hived off into a metaphysical box labelled 'divine otherness', is part of our general human capacity to imagine states of existence which are different from those immediately presented to us by our senses.

The mental impression which each one of us has about the nature of the world-out-there is the result of a computation process in which mental representations are generated out of the signals which flow into the brain through our senses and are then interpreted in the light of experience and prior anticipation. But we are also capable of generating 'imaginary' representations which are quite independent of any immediate sensory inputs. The fact that we can do this has probably been very important for human evolution, for it gives members of the genus *Homo* enormous competitive advantages as compared with less adaptable genera.

Man's superiority over other creatures is manifested in his greater adaptability. Most animals are tightly adapted to a particular environmental niche; man has learnt how to modify himself and his environment artificially so as to be able to exist almost anywhere, even at the bottom of the sea or on the surface of the moon. The essential feature of the intelligence that enables man to do these things consists of a unique capacity for making operationally effective guesses about the circumstances that may be encountered in unfamiliar situations. We have developed this capacity as a part of our social nature. We live in societies in which not only our own individual behaviour is unpredictable but every other individual's behaviour is equally unpredictable; yet in practice we are able to cope with this unpredictability.

The essence of this coping is that we play a game of 'as if': we plan our strategies of social chess on the assumption that things are much simpler than they really are. We pretend that the unfamiliar is familiar and act accordingly. To this end, the man-made world in which human beings conduct their lives is always radically simplified as compared with the 'natural' environment. Our houses are constructed out of a simplified geometry of straight lines and circles; our preferred categories are binary – black/white, yes/no. That part of experience which doesn't fit in with this drastic simplifying process is discarded as a residue; it is declared to be 'unnatural', 'metaphysical', 'part of the other world'. It is part of the game that whenever we are being rational and practical we should carefully avoid any recognition of this 'other' part of our experience.

Mind you, non-rational emotions break out into the open from time to time, and it is probably very important that they should. It is significant that nearly all human societies have devised complex social institutions which provide tidy channels through which suppressed topics of a sexual, scatological, 'supernatural' kind can be legitimately discussed, in emasculated form, under the guise of joking. But joking is an escape-valve abnormality the very existence of which reinforces our belief that the normal social world should be orderly and comprehensible.

From this it follows that everything that is incomprehensible comes to be treated as dangerous, off-stage, 'power', which threatens the natural order of things.

Normality, Abnormality and the Pursuit of Salvation

The verbal oppositions living/dead, human/divine, natural/supernatural are, on the face of it, clear-cut alternatives, either-or, not both at once. That would imply that our contrived distinction between normal and abnormal is equally clear-cut, which is, no doubt, how we should like it to be.

But the bridge-building of religious ideology tends to blur the edges of this tidy intellectual construction. It creates ambiguous abnormal entities which are neither one thing nor the other: virgin-mothers, god-men, reincarnate ancestors. This is logically inevitable. Since the other world is specified in the first place as a zone of abnormality, it must follow that any human being who achieves any kind of abnormal physical state is already halfway to achieving the status of a divine being in the other world.

So we are faced with a paradox. If we aspire to be perfect as men the desirable goal is rational normality, but if we desire to come closer to God then the goal should be abnormality.

In religious, as contrasted with secular, ideology this distinction is explicit, and both ethnography and history reveal a great variety of techniques for the achievement of the appropriate abnormal physical states. They consist in pushing things to extremes in one or other of two possible directions. One direction is that of asceticism which entails the repudiation of all normal appetites – sex, food, drink, movement, conversation; in myth, the ultimate yogi whose very placidity is so unnatural that its power can potentially destroy the universe is Śiva sitting cross-legged in the Himalayas contemplating his erect penis through all eternity. The early Christian hermits of the Sinai desert sought sainthood and divine power by very similar methods, e.g. St Simeon Stylites who sat on top of a pillar for forty years.

In religions dominated by an ascetic ideology all 'feeling', that is all uncontrolled response to the senses, is treated as sin, a contaminating influence of the 'illusory' experience of this world (e.g. the Buddhist concept of *maya*). By freeing ourselves of sensory responses we shall be able to enter the reality of the other world, which is the form of experience otherwise reserved for those who are already dead.

St Simeon Stylites – a still from Luis Buñuel's film *Simon of the Desert*.

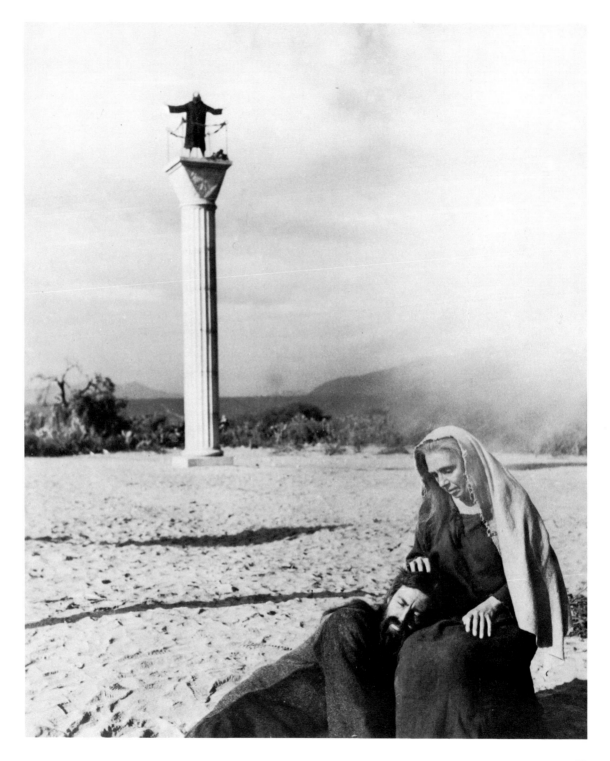

The other route to abnormality is by way of ecstasy. Sensual experience is valued for its own sake; contrivances of all sorts are employed to intensify sensory appetites beyond the limits of normality; in myth, the motionless yogi is replaced by dancing Śiva, or Śiva in eternal sexual congress with the irresistible Parvātī.

In the simpler societies, as we can observe them today, the pursuit of salvation through asceticism is very rare, while the route through ecstasy is very common. I would suppose that this has always been the case.

The devices which may be employed to heighten sensibility by way of the ecstatic mode depend upon cultural tradition. Stimulants and hallucinatory drugs in great variety have been used since time immemorial in all parts of the world, but often in combination with more mechanical procedure. The object of the exercise is to achieve a state of cataleptic trance, or at least a condition in which the conscious Ego begins to feel himself dissociated from his physical body and no longer fully in control of what that body is doing.

Most of the mechanical, sensation-generating procedures employed in ecstatic religious cults of this kind have their counterparts in the fun fairs of the contemporary Western World. The commonest involve violent and prolonged dancing and very loud music, but we also meet with psychedelic lights, terrors in the dark, giant swings and so on. In Sabah I have seen a whole congregation of more than twenty individuals achieve a trance condition by jumping rhythmically on a kind of trampoline floor having a vertical oscillation of about 8 feet. The extraordinary tortures to which ecstatic devotees very often subject themselves – fire-walking, driving skewers through parts of the body, self-imposed bodily mutilations, acts of animal-like savagery – serve the double function of demonstrating that the individual concerned really is in an abnormal psychophysical condition and of providing a reinforcement which enhances the condition as such.

In these performances the particular type of sensual experience – the swinging, the dancing, the din, the drug-induced hallucination, the torture, the symptom of bestiality etc. – is not valued as an end in itself but as a means to an end. The sensual experience, as such, is simply an indication of the presence of power. Judgment as to whether the power is good (e.g. that of saints and deities) or bad (e.g. that of witches and demons) is a matter of cultural convention but there are no grounds for supposing that, in general, the medium 'enjoys' his ecstatic experience. Ecstasy is pursued as a religious duty rather than as a means to private indulgence.

In the context of such cults dogma asserts that a condition of trance indicates a dissociation of the 'soul' from its ordinary material body. In this abnormal condition the shaman/medium is both alive and dead, a being who provides a bridge between the here-and-now and the other. In such conditions the soul of the entranced medium may visit the other world or, alternatively, the body of the medium may temporarily become a vehicle possessed by a spirit from the other world.

Despite the similarity of means and (presumably) also the similarity of sensual

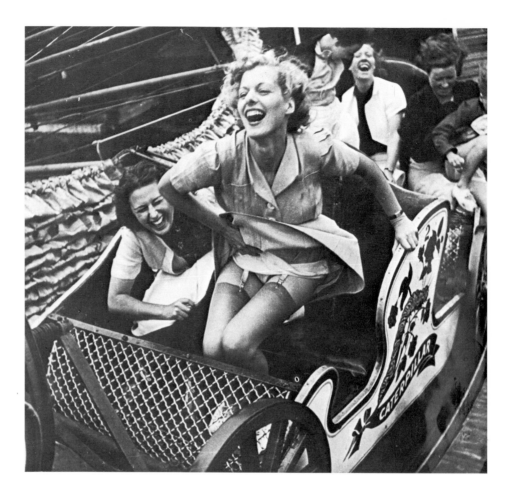

experience, cult behaviour of this kind, which has a deep religious basis, needs to be distinguished from the private pursuit of hallucinatory experience for its own sake which has had such a vogue in the youth culture of Western society over the past twenty years. Shamans are neither hedonists nor sybarites, nor are they trying to explore untrodden fields of sensory experience. On the contrary, like the priests and hermits of ascetic religions, they are conforming to a precisely predetermined ritual code.

Literacy and the cult of rationality

Underlying the argument of the previous sections are several related propositions which need to be spelled out. The first is plain enough: in all religious cults the abnormal is valued above the normal because it is supposed that only by achieving a

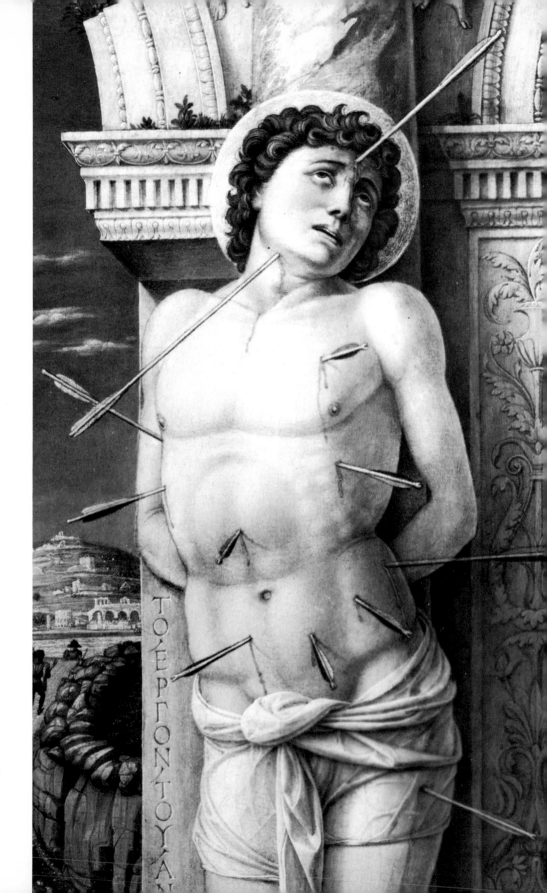

Detail from Andrea Mantegna's painting *St Sebastian*, c. 1457.

Opposite: the Japanese writer Yukio Mishima posing as St Sebastian in 1970. A few months later he took his life in public by committing hara kiri.

100

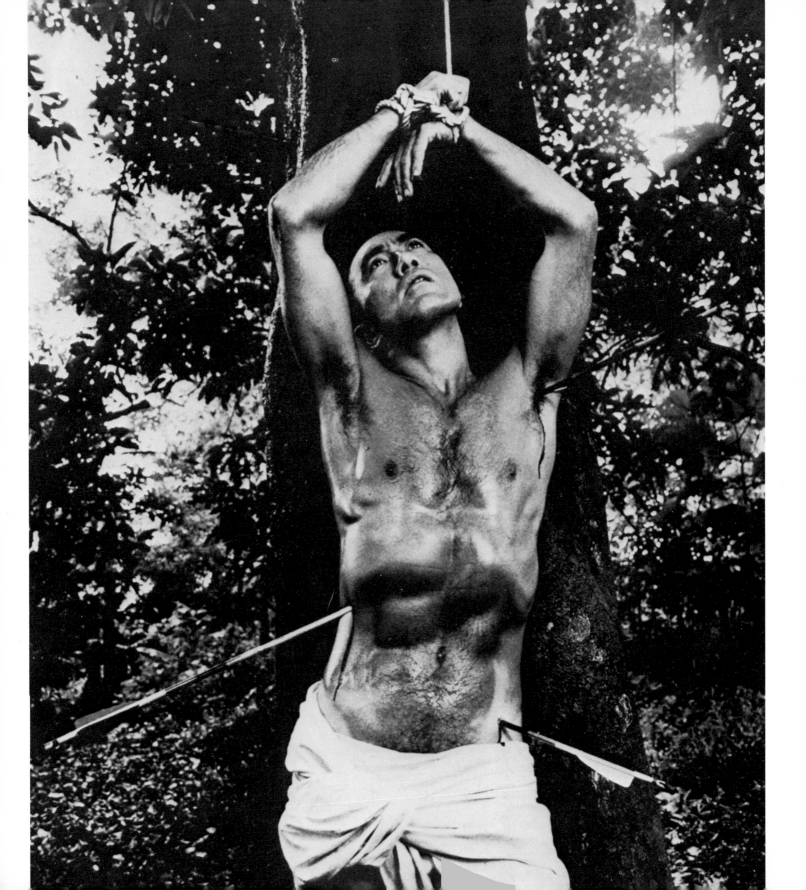

condition of abnormality can we hope to gain access to the potency which is otherwise the exclusive perquisite of beings of the other world.

The second theme is perhaps less clear. In the jargon of this essay I am saying that the idea of deity, considered as an external potency influencing the affairs of living men, is a paradigm for two other ideas from which it is verbally distinguished, that of survival after death and that of a separable immortal soul (*psyche*), which is treated as the source of the living individual's internal potency.

My third theme, which I have so far hardly developed, is supplementary to the second. I suggest that we misrepresent religion if we separate out its component elements and serve them up as a syntagmatic chain linked together by metonymy, yet that is precisely what we always tend to do. Just as our total sensory experience becomes impoverished when we analyse our sensual responses fragment by fragment, so also the literary, rational, ascetic tradition of the Western world emasculates religion by dismembering its total ideology into separate themes, so that God becomes one concept, survival after death another, and man's immortal soul a third. As a case in point E. R. Dodds, in a celebrated book about ancient Greek religion published in 1951, working from literary sources rather than intuition, persuades himself that these are three quite separate ideas, separately developed, one after another. Which is all very nice and tidy for the purpose of a rational literary description of irrational behaviour, but no religion was ever like that.

So let me go back to the beginning and say a bit more about this business of totalization versus fragmentation, paradigms versus syntagms, metaphors versus metonymy, and the relevance of all these dyads for our apprehension of the connections between sensory experience and rational analysis.

Any form of written script is syntagmatic in construction. Egyptian hieroglyphics, Assyrian cuneiform, Chinese ideograms, alphabetic scripts of all kinds, break down into elemental units (letters, radicals etc.) which do not contain meaning in themselves but acquire meaning when strung together into syntagmatic chains: 'C A T spells cat.' Those who communicate with one another in writing thus have a strong built-in bias towards analysis. And the more widespread the use of literacy as a standard mode of communication the more 'rational' and analytic the whole society becomes. Anyone who communicates information by means of writing must take his ideas to pieces before he writes them down; and when he does write them down the ideas come out one after another in a logical sequence and are *not* all superimposed as in the confusion of a palimpsest.

It is not, of course, the case that all written discourse is strictly rational, but rational argument, narrowly defined, is only likely to emerge in a context of literacy.

In non-literate societies, verbal knowledge (in the form of legend, tradition, magical spells and religious myth) always has a context of performance – singing, dancing, music, sacrificial rite. What is said in words is simply an incomplete paradigm for what is also being acted out in other ways. All the different senses are brought into play; the muses are a team; Clio (history) does not act on her own. But

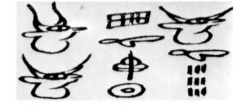

Pictographic script (dating from the 19th century) of the Moso people of south-west China, showing prayers and invocations.

the literary man typically works by himself in private, 'putting his thoughts on paper'; in such circumstances the role of sensuality can be (and usually is) reduced to an absolute minimum.

This, I suggest, explains how it comes about that the intellectual attitude which is characteristically proclaimed as scholarly and correct by most educated people in the Western world is precisely the opposite of that which I have outlined above in exemplifying the pursuit of salvation by way of ecstasy. Not only is normality consistently valued above abnormality, but asceticism is treated as rational and normal while ecstasy is despised and classed as irrational and abnormal. This transformation from a non-literate to a literate context can be expressed in diagrammatic form, thus:

1 *Non-literate context*: predominance of metaphor depending upon paradigmatic associations; subjective sensory experience treated as a synchronic unity as in musical harmony.

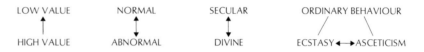

2 *Literate context*: predominance of metonymy depending upon causally linked syntagmatic sequences; isolated sensory signals treated as indices of objective 'facts', out there, which add up to a diachronic unity as in musical melody.

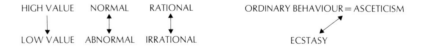

Historically, the most striking examples of the dominance of ascetic over ecstatic religious values have occurred in literate settings in Buddhist, Hindu, Moslem and Christian cultures. The vow of silence and the lifelong commitment to sexual abstinence characteristic of many monastic and eremitic institutions is commonly associated with great reverence for sacred texts. The idea seems to be that those who would come near to God through close study of the Book must be deprived of all distracting sensual contact with the world of men. In many parts of Islam the proper career for a blind male child is to become a Mullah. He cannot *see* the text of the Koran, so he must learn it off by heart from beginning to end. In that purely verbal, internalized form, the word of God is free from all human corruption. But devotion to sacred texts is not confined to avowed adherents of the major religions; in contemporary Christendom it is the secular political fanatics who most frequently behave like blind Mullahs.

Sensory combinations and transformations

Because of the metonymic ascetic assumptions that are built into our literary education, nearly all readers of this essay are likely to take it for granted that our senses are separable and that each separate sense corresponds to a separate sensory experience. We use our eyes to see, our ears to hear, our nose to smell, our tongue to taste, our fingers to touch, and so on. But apart from reading there are not many kinds of completely monosensual experiences. In the major loci of sensuality which are, for all human beings, eating, sex, defecation and the fear of death, the 'separate' senses are all loaded on top of one another, as in metaphor; the object of love is good to see, good to touch, good to smell, good to hear, good to taste. Moreover, the loci themselves are muddled up. As Lévi-Strauss has perceptively argued, there is a near-universal tendency in the iconography of myth and of visual symbolism to transform experiences which belong to the field of sex and procreation into experience relating to eating, vomiting, defecation, and sometimes *vice versa*.

The gentry class of pre-revolutionary China was one of the few societies known to history in which cooking had been developed into a fine art. As in contemporary France it was felt to be entirely polite to discuss at table the precise details of the food one was eating and its mode of preparation. Chinese *haute cuisine* of this sort was still in vogue in West China when I myself was living in Szechwan around 1934. Despite the corruptions of taste that resulted from my Western upbringing I had no great difficulty in appreciating the merits of such delicacies as unborn mice and Szechwan white fungus, but my scale of evaluations was quite different from that of my hosts. Nearly all *their* distinctions were based on the supposed aphrodisiac qualities of the various dishes!

Because the ascetic values of Christianity have made gluttony as well as fornication a deadly sin we in the West are almost as reluctant to discuss in public the details of the pleasures of eating as we are those of copulation, and because of such taboos we commonly refuse to recognize the harmonic echoes of sensual experience. Yet our pretence that the various senses have separate spheres of activity, from some of which the dangerous topics of sex and religion can be excluded simply by a careful choice of words, is highly artificial. Small details of our verbal usages give the show away. The word 'scent' with its suggestion of a civet cat on heat has now been converted by the media men into 'perfume', but we still use the word 'taste' as if it were an all-embracing type of feeling covering every aspect of aesthetic appreciation.

The paradox in this essay is that, if my argument is valid, it will not be understood. Feeling is a total experience; we become conscious because of messages that reach the brain through the eyes, ears, nose, mouth, fingers, stomach, genitals. . . . But these messages are alternative simultaneous metaphors of one and the same world out there; we do not end up with separate constructions, a sight world, a sound world, a smell world and so on. All is transformation. Even as I write, 'messages' appropriate to the auditory channel of communication are being converted to tactile images which will generate responses through the eyes. Yet to 'understand' this sensual confusion we must take it to pieces and consider one thing at a time. If we do that, we shall lose the sense of totality; but if we do not do that, we shall not understand.

Evidence from the study of animal behaviour and from comparative ethnography indicates that the mental capacities which man originally developed in response to the environmental circumstances of his pre-human existence during the hominid phase of his evolution are now greatly under-used. But the machinery is still there which could provide us all with an eidetic memory of perfect recall.

We are fortunate that most of us are not burdened with memory of that sort, and we are likewise fortunate that most of our other sensory capabilities are dormant rather than active for most of the time. The reason why we can get along without making much use of most of our sensory capabilities is that we have language. Language is uniquely an attribute of man; language makes man what he is; language makes redundant many of the capacities which man developed along with other animals during the pre-human phase of his evolution. Not only that, but the efficient use of language *requires* that these other capacities be *not* utilized. But language is syntagmatic, sequential.

The world that is accessible to our senses is a continuum. If our experiences of that world consisted solely of superimposed flat screen-images generated by our senses of sight, hearing and smell, as is presumably the case for many varieties of animal, there would be no need to break up that experience into 'things' at all. Our human preference for segmentation and classification (which allows us to perceive the world as a causally linked chain of separate parts rather than as a unified, simultaneously felt total experience) is directly tied in with our use of language. For language itself is a chain linkage of morphemes (words) and it can only adequately represent the world if the world is felt to be structured in the same way.

In order to transform the continuous simultaneous world of sense experience into the discontinuous, sequential, chain-linked world of verbal description we must drastically simplify perception. We must suppress all conscious recognition of the logical interstices that lie between the 'things' that we are prepared to recognize, and we must pretend that all the resultant entities, however diverse they may 'really' be, fit tidily into the very limited number of slots provided by our verbal categories. For example, all human beings must be either male or female; they are not allowed to be betwixt and between. So when our senses tell us that large numbers of human individuals behave as if they *were* betwixt and between we escape from our dilemma in one of three ways:

1   we refuse to recognize the facts (the topic becomes taboo);
2   we resort to joking to invalidate the implication of the facts, and then treat them with ridicule;
3   we declare the facts to be supernatural, and then treat them with awe.

The principle is very general and applies to all categories of experience which fall outside the verbal slots which we are prepared to recognize as 'normal'.

In our society verbal normality equates with 'rational'. The rational world is that which can be made to appear orderly by means of the use of words or mathematical equations. Everything else is irrational.

Since books are written in words and do not carry supplementary signals such as smell or noise or temperature, any book which is to be understood (including this one) must conform to the normal canons of rationality as specified above. Conversely the category 'irrational' embraces all channels of communication which are both non-verbal and non-literate.

The principal sub-categories of this wide-ranging residue are (i) all non-verbal noise, including the ordered types of noise which we rate as music; (ii) dancing, including combat games such as football; (iii) painting, sculpture, architecture, the plastic arts of all kinds; (iv) odours, both natural and synthetic; (v) the taste of food; (vi) sexual intercourse in all its degrees. These of course are precisely the prototype symbols by which the puritan characterizes luxury and vice.

If we reduce this whole argument to a sequential history it comes out roughly as follows:

In primitive pre-literate societies there is no systematic distinction between the rational and the irrational. There is, however, a distinction in social time: normal time is devoted to secular activities in which rational behaviour predominates over irrational behaviour; abnormal time is devoted to sacred activities in which irrational behaviour predominates over rational behaviour. The pursuit of irrational sensual experience is treated as a means of gaining access to supernatural power and of moving social time forward into the next phase. As in literate societies, secular time alternates with sacred time: holy days are holidays.

In advanced literate societies there is a systematic distinction between the rational and the irrational. The technological and scientific advances that have taken place in these societies since the end of the fifteenth century are directly linked with the spread of book-learning and the consequent (and necessary) denigration of the irrational. The universal technological and political ascendancy of the literate societies over their pre-literate neighbours is the consequence of rational economic and political decision-making. The suppression of redundant emotion is a necessary part of such thinking. If we do not treat 'unnecessary' sensual experience as a luxury, technological and scientific progress will be impossible. It requires a climate of asceticism to generate such attitudes. A rational society must reduce its artists to critics; there is no room for poets in the laboratory.

All of which was said much more clearly by Giambattista Vico just 250 years ago:

> ...and human nature, so far as it is like that of animals, carries with it this property, that the senses are its sole way of knowing things. Hence poetic wisdom, the first

wisdom of the gentile world, must have begun with a metaphysics not rational and abstract like that of learned men now, but felt and imagined as that of these first men must have been, who, without power of ratiocination, were all robust sense and vigorous imagination. This metaphysics was their poetry, a faculty born with them; born of their ignorance of causes. . . . Their poetry was at first divine, because . . . they imagined the causes of the things they felt . . . to be gods. . . . In such fashion the first men of the gentile nations, children of nascent mankind, created things according to their own ideas.*

But we cannot go back to the Garden of Eden.

* Vico, *Scienza Nuova*, 1744 edition, Book II, Section 1, Chapter 1, Bergin & Fisch (1968) translation, pp. 116–17.

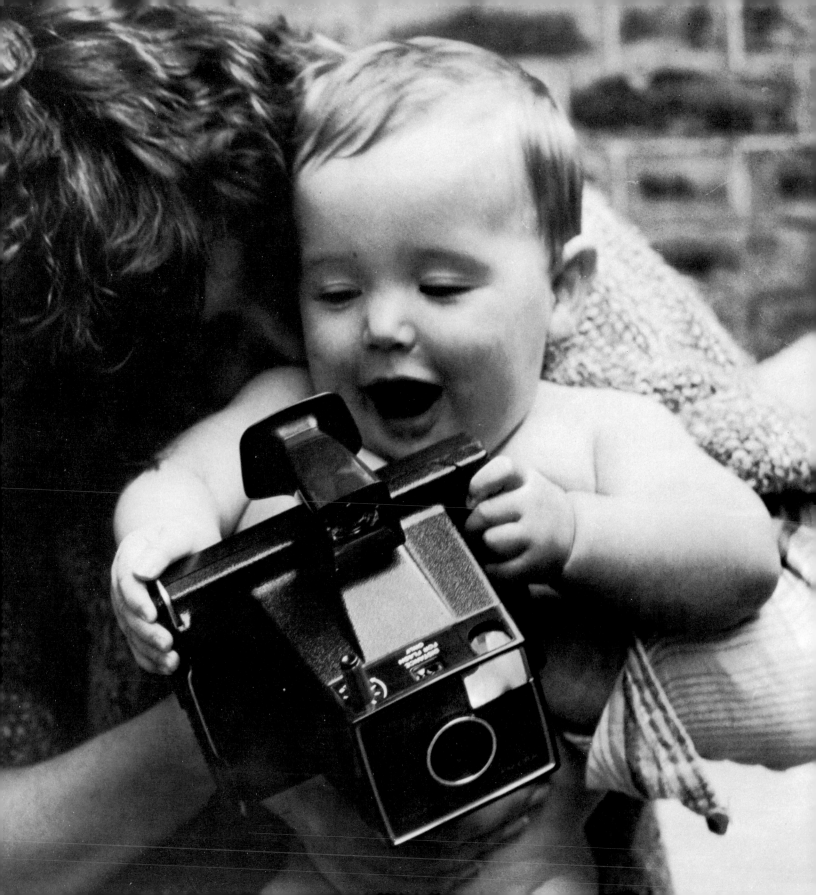

EDMUND CARPENTER

Edmund Carpenter has been described as America's foremost 'anthropologist of the senses'. His books include *Eskimo Realities, They Became What They Beheld,* and *Oh, What a Blow That Phantom Gave Me!*

They became what they beheld

The senses aren't mere input channels: they make their own worlds of spaces and relations. Every sense has its own paradigm of pleasure and pain, creates its own time and space – is, in fact, a unique environment. Similarly, each medium has its bias, creates its environment, produces its effects. Media interpenetrate and interplay with one another, much as senses do. But the bias of each can be isolated and its effects, achieved separately or in combination with other media, can be studied. Media, like art forms, are models of sensory programming. Remove an organ from a body and the remaining organs play new roles; add an organ and reorganization also occurs. This is true of media as well: new media recast old media in new roles. The appearance of television, for example, forced all other media to play new roles: radio brought back 'theatre in the round', classroom seats were unscrewed from the floor, and we all became 'wired for sound'.

For 2500 years, under literacy, Western civilization was dominated by one medium: language. All truth, it was believed, could be housed inside its walls. Writers attempted to enclose the sum of human experience within the walls of rational discourse; scientists attempted to order reality within the governance of language. Non-verbal media became subservient to verbal categories.

But the synthesis of understanding which once made common speech possible, today no longer works. As George Steiner points out, large areas of meaning are now ruled by non-verbal languages such as mathematics or symbolic logic or film. Little or nothing is 'verbal' in modern music or art. Both are languages, yet nothing can be said about either that is pertinent to the traditional habits of linguistic sense. Absolutely nothing can be said about a Franz Kline painting. A De Kooning canvas has no subject of which one can render a verbal account; it bypasses language and seems to play directly on our nerve ends. 'Whereof one cannot speak,' writes Wittgenstein, 'thereof one must be silent.'

The same applies to much contemporary dance, film and music, especially electronic music. When we ask the contemporary artist to explain himself, he refers us back to his work. He's reluctant to translate his effort into words, that is, into a wholly different medium. 'If I could tell you what it meant,' said Isadora Duncan, 'there would be no point in dancing it.'

One cannot translate modern mathematics into words. One cannot even paraphrase. The two are independent systems of notation. This applies to other

109

media as well. To copyright music, one publishes it, but much contemporary music cannot be recorded visually. It is its own language: 'A baby crying in the night/In no language but a cry.'

The monopoly, even tyranny, language enjoyed under literacy was shattered by electricity. Language was once the sole, or at least dominant, actor on stage. Today the stage is crowded. No medium dominates the others. All are free to develop into languages of their own, as articulate and elaborate as those of verbal discourse.

'. . . to go on from there, I can't use words; they don't say enough. . . .' – Jefferson Airplane.

We might liken it to the difference between synchronized music played by musicians obedient to a strict conductor and music with interweaving rhythm patterns played by improvisors, each with his own downbeat. Certain African musicians carry on five simultaneous rhythms, the melody, handclapping and tapping the feet; the individual performs all three simultaneously, though not in synchronization. Most literate men, conditioned to take one thing at a time, simply cannot do that. But post-literate men can. The gap between generations is a gap between sensory profiles.

Electronic media have eroded traditional individualism, weakened representative government and led to a general loss of those freedoms and protections enjoyed under literacy. The ballot-box can't create images for the electronic world. Freedom has shifted from government to art. Today's varied media, each a unique codification of reality, offer range and depth for human expression and fulfilment perhaps equal to those abandoned. Man used tools to unlock the resources of the earth. Now he uses language and art to unlock resources within himself. Mating a language or an art with electricity creates new media of astronomical power. These media aren't toys: they shouldn't be in the hands of Peter Pan executives. They can be entrusted only to new artists, because they are art forms.

'Oh, what a beautiful baby!' 'That's nothing,' replied the mother, 'you should see his photograph.'

California hippie: '. . . one couple I know rarely speak but share the same rhythms with tamborines and drums, as well as with their breathing. These rhythms are the same as the ones their electric fan and refrigerator make.'

Billy Graham reports a higher percentage of converts on closed-circuit TV than among those watching him 'live'.

For five hundred years, print culture depressed all sensory life except sight. Literate man called painters, poets, and musicians 'artists', but cooks, gardeners and hairdressers were seldom more than servants. Appearance became everything. Fashion was concerned only with sight. Fashion models looked like manikins: the clothes, not the girl, mattered. 'Clothes make the man.' Visual values became the mark of civilized man as compared to the values of the barbarian. Eroticism was

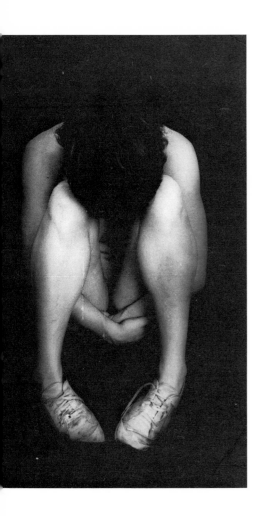

almost entirely visual. Men became 'girl-watchers', peeping toms. Literacy produced the pin-up, the Sweater Girl and 'falsies', all of which survive now as camp. Today, when lovemaking is primarily by touch and smell, the *Playboy* nude appears as remote as sculpture.

Alienation from all senses save sight led to emotional detachment – the inability to feel and express emotions. Literate man not only concealed emotions, he experienced them less: 'Unmoved, cold and to temptation slow.' Psychiatrists tell us that people who can express emotions can more readily experience them and that those who cannot express themselves are ill. In tribal societies especially, perception or cognition is associated with, or immediately followed by, an 'emotion'. Every idea is not only a state of knowing but a tendency to movement: 'To see her is to love her'; 'I shuddered at the thought.' Emotion affects both heart and lungs. 'Every emotion quickens the action of the heart and with it the respiration,' observed Darwin. 'When a fearful object is before us we pant and cannot deeply inspire.'

Emotion tends to beget bodily motion. In Homer, the manliest warriors wept openly, beat their chests, tore their hair, and when this was sung about in the Athenian markets, it's probable that listeners joined in the expression of these emotions. Hearing these accounts meant experiencing them. But one can read them without emotion. Any newspaper front page is a mass of tragedies, yet we read unmoved. We could never act or dance such tragedies without emotion. Nor sing them. Nor express them as poetry. But reading is different. Silent reading is thinking deserted by emotion. It leads to a high degree of separation of mental concepts from the plurality of the concrete. 'Normal' readers don't get emotionally involved in what they read. They enjoy a sensory detachment – an ability to act without reacting. But printed news may turn on an 'unbalanced' reader. Accounts of hotel fires may lead to more fires. Oswald, Ray, Sirhan – each saved and pocketed newspaper clippings.

No environment is perceptible because it saturates the whole field of attention. One can perceive it only after alienation – after some degree of alienation. I can swallow the saliva in my mouth because it's 'me', but I can't swallow it if I put it first into a glass. So long as I transact with my environment – my ecological whole – I can't perceive it; it doesn't even environ me. It's an extension of me. And I can't smell myself.

Early analysts were called 'alienists'. Alienation begins when one feels revulsion with one's body, and fears the sensate world. Trudie Shoop, the dancer, helped schizophrenics rediscover themselves by re-teaching them the earliest movements of childhood.

When primitives talk about their own world, they speak about how things smell, taste, feel, sound: toes gripping roots along a slippery bank; peppery food burning the rectum: 'It is pleasant,' said a Vedda, 'for us to feel the rain beating over our shoulders, and good to go out and dig yams, and come home wet, and see the fire burning in the cave, and sit around it.' Consider the Eskimo who, with visibility zero, navigates his kayak rapidly along dangerous coastlines, guided by the feel of wind and smell of fog, by sounds of surf and nesting birds, and particularly by the feel of the pattern of waves and current against his buttocks. With such interplay of the senses, there can be no isolation of one sense. A hunter who relied on sight alone would return empty-handed; a traveller who ignored odours and winds and sounds would soon be lost. The lone Eskimo traveller often dozes on his sled, facing away from the wind, his parka hood all but closed. But the fur of the parka, brushing against his face, warns him of wind changes, and he rouses himself, checks how the wind is cutting into snow drifts, signals changes to the dogs if necessary, and then sinks back into light sleep.

A child learns to separate the senses when he learns, in class, to read silently. His legs twist, he bites his tongue, but by an enormous *tour de force* he learns to fragment his senses, to turn on one at a time and keep the others in neutral. And so he is indoctrinated into that literate world where readers seek silent solitude, concert-goers close their eyes, and gallery guards warn, 'Don't touch!'

Not long ago when some British children were asked, 'What are the twelve loveliest things you know?' one boy answered:

> The cold of ice cream.
> The scrunch of leaves.
> The feel of clean cloze.
> Water running into a bath.
> Cold wind on a hot day.
> Climbing up a hill looking down.
> Hot water bottle in bed.
> Honey in your mouth.
> Smell in a drug store.
> Babies smiling.
> The feeling inside when you sing.
> Baby kittens.

A little girl's list went:

> Our dog's eyes.
> Street lights on the river.
> Wet stones.
> The smell of rain.
> An organ playing.
> Red roofs in trees.
> Smoke rising.
> Rain on your cheeks.
> The smell of cut grass.

Red velvet.
The smell of picnic teas.
The moon in clouds.

'Work' means specialism. It equals fragmented tasks and consequent non-involvement of the whole person. Play equals involvement, as in hobbies or conversation. Where involvement is low, work is high. Tribal man doesn't work, hence has no need for leisure, no need to recreate his whole self. His whole self is already totally involved in living.

Dreams, myths, rituals are all forms of total involvement. The dreamer divests himself of private identity and unites with the corporate image of his group. Tribal Africans are reported to require less sleep than literate wage-earners. The nine-to-five African civil servant needs eight hours' sleep, though his physical labour is minimal. What he requires is dreaming. Apparently dreaming is mandatory for human life. Literate man, in dreams, is able to suspend temporarily the unbearable strain of individual identity: he can efface himself by merging with cosmic forces. Tribal man requires less night-dreaming because he achieves this corporate identification through daytime rituals, myths, art, language. We're re-entering the tribal world, but this time we're going through the tribal dance and drama wide awake.

Palaeolithic man worked in the darkness of caverns, his paintings illuminated by flickering torch: elusive images appeared/disappeared. His art emerged as a direct response to inner light. He employed 'the inward eye', and he had no concept of three-dimensional perspective with a vanishing point in the distance before him. For him, the vanishing point was within himself and he went through it by stepping into his art.

Hans Arp drew his curved, interpenetrating lines, which so closely resemble certain Palaeolithic drawings, with half-closed eyes: ' . . . under lowered lids, the inner movement streams untainted to the hand. In a darkened room it is easier to follow the guidance of the inner movement than in the open air. A conductor of inner music, the great designer of prehistoric images, worked with eyes turned upwards. So his drawings gain in transparency; open to penetration, to sudden inspiration, to recovery of the inner melody, to the circling approach; and the whole is transmuted into one great exhalation.' This is the inward quest, the search for meaning beyond the world of appearances; it's the 'prophet blinded so that sight is yielded for insight.'

Coleridge, De Quincey, Baudelaire, Rimbaud used drugs to dislocate perception and reorganize their imaginative lives. They wanted to get out of the boundaries and patterns of perception as they experienced it in their own culture in order to discover new images. They all had the ambition to discover new worlds of perception, new worlds of sensibility. In many tribes the youth seeking insight goes apart from his fellows and lives for a time in the wilderness, fasting and praying. 'If he is the proper sort, he will return with a message from the god he set out to seek, but even if he fails in that particular, he will have had a vision or seen a marvel – and these are always worth listening to and thinking about.'

When tribal people tell of such experiences, they rarely mention things seen. They refer to experiences felt, to 'inner voices'. Clearly, such experiences aren't primarily visual. Insight is more appropriate than 'vision'; 'hearer' or 'feeler' is more accurate than 'seer'.

Primitive people generally regard the eye as both transmitter and receiver. Many hold that a luminous quality goes from the eye into what it sees. Village Greeks today openly stare: they want to look you in the eye, in the same way they openly eavesdrop! All reject you by not wanting to see or hear you. In early Greek, 'to look at' meant to breathe at; 'perceiving' meant taking in. 'Check thy dread eye and the blasts of thy breath,' warns Euripides. Plato believed sight was the result of 'fusion of rays, the light of the eyes flowing out some distance into the kindred air and the light from objects meeting it'. Such theories had their analogy with children who equate seeing and giving light. For very young children, seeing is partly outside the eye. It comes from the eye, it gives light, and they're puzzled why they don't feel it. Boy of five: 'Daddy, why don't our looks mix when they meet?'

No handier illustration exists than comic books. Superman's heat vision can paralyse an enemy, penetrate concrete, melt a safe, cook a hot dog. When his look meets Superwoman's look, a flash occurs at the point of impact.

The notion that looking is a generative force, that the meeting of two looks can be creative, is widespread. According to Freud, blindness symbolizes castration; hence blinded Oedipus leans on a stick, the stick being a phallic symbol. The Bambara of Africa say it's by the eyes, as well as the sexual organs, that a wife is united to her husband during intercourse. Defective children, they say, are those conceived during intercourse when the eyes are closed. One is reminded of the Hindu tale of the man who offended a god and in punishment was so ugly that his wife kept her eyes closed during intercourse, as a result of which their child was born blind.

Until the seventeenth century, the Western world thought of the eye as a broadcasting station, a centre of diffusion and emanation from the pupil or the 'apple of the eye'. The psalmist's 'Keep me in your eye' meant: Keep me in existence, God; don't let me off your radar screen. 'Laid eyes on' meant to call into existence; 'overlook' was a verb associated with the evil eye. The eye was assumed to be the organ of action, the ear the organ of reception. Gradually, under literacy, the sense ratios altered and the eye came to be regarded as a means of passive pickup of experience. That trend has suddenly been reversed: the ancient notion that the eye is an organ of power is once more being expressed.

In the tribal world, the most powerful force radiating from any being is believed to be breath, which is regarded as life itself. God 'breathed into his nostrils the breath of

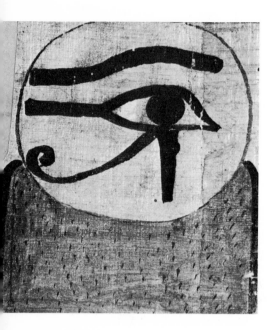

The eye of Ra, from *The Book of the Dead*, c. 1000 BC.

114

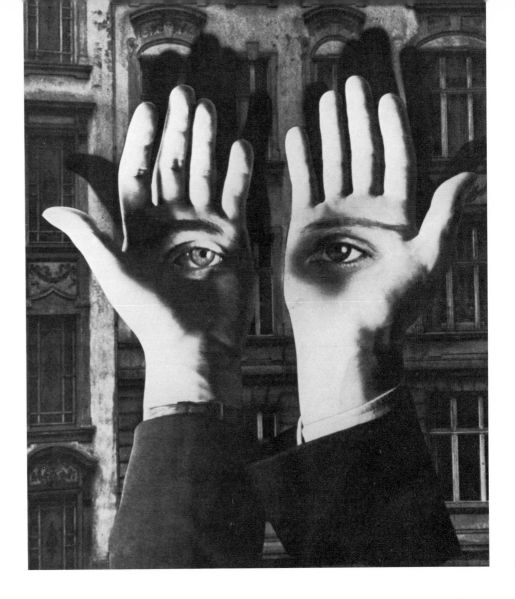

life, and man became a living soul'. In such societies, to speak means to call into being: 'And God said, Let there be light; and there was light'; 'By the word of the Lord were the Heavens made, and all the hosts of them by the breath of his mouth.' In Eskimo, the word 'to make poetry' is the word 'to breathe'; both are derivations of *anerca*, the soul, that which is eternal, the breath of life.

Since the essence of a thing was thought to be its flavour, its aroma, to experience that essence directly meant taking it into oneself. One became what one ate. The word 'taste' itself originally had a much broader meaning than simply gastronomic experience. It meant to explore, to test: 'Tasted the waye' (1480); 'The men of armes entre into the dykes, and tasted the dykes with their speares, and passed over to the fote of the wall' (1525). It also meant to have carnal knowledge of: 'You have tasted

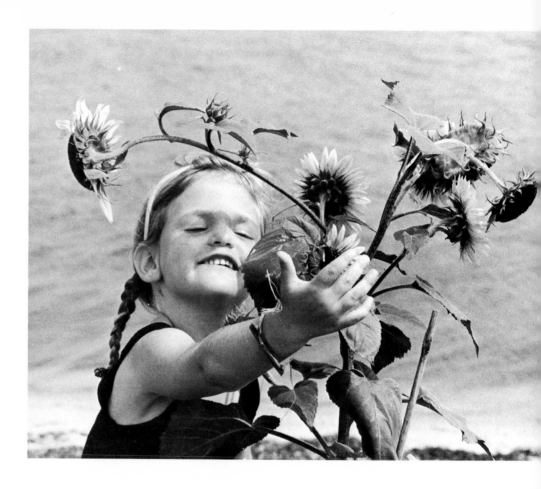

her in bed' (*Cymbeline*, II. iv.); 'What, see, talk, touch, nay taste her!' (1752). To be 'out of taste' meant to be unable to distinguish flavours. 'True to taste' meant the sense of what is appropriate, harmonious, beautiful. Children often explore by tasting. So do many primitives. In Flaherty's *Nanook of the North*, Nanook examines a strange phonograph record by listening, seeing, touching, tasting. Lovers find each other 'good enough to eat'.

The concept of an essence radiating out from an inner source applies to the other senses as well. Plutarch warned that not only fiery rays darting from the eyes, but the voice, breath and odour as well could harm, or aid. Andaman Islanders paint themselves with clay to deny their odours to evil spirits. Arabs consistently breathe on friends when they talk: 'To smell one's friend is not only nice but desirable'; to deny him your breath is to deny him yourself. Chuckchee of Siberia greet each other by sniffing down the back of the neck. In the jungles of the Andamans, each flower period is thought to possess its own kind of force, of which the scent is the manifest sign and the fruit is the product. When a girl reaches puberty, she blossoms, as it were, the later ripening being the birth of her children. Like the jungle plants, she is believed to be under the influence of generative forces which everywhere produce blossoming and fruiting. She is therefore named after that particular odoriferous plant in flower when she reaches her blossoming time. Certain remedies possess strong odours: Andamanese either eat them or breathe in their vapours; such odours, they say, effect cures.

Literate man regards silence as empty of value. He calls radio silence 'dead air' and condemns any cocktail party marked by long silences. Silence in music is often interrupted by applause from someone who mistakenly thinks the concert is over. Writing of the Bedouin tribesmen, T. E. Lawrence tells how one of them took him through a deserted palace where each room had a different scent, and then called, 'Come and smell the very sweetest scent of all' and led him to a gaping window where the empty wind of the desert went throbbing past. 'This,' he told him, 'is the best: it has no taste.'

Not to speak doesn't mean one has nothing to say. Those who don't may be brimming over with emotions which can be expressed only in gesture and play of features. Gestures convey inner emotions which would still remain unexpressed when everything that can be told has been told and words 'get in the way.' Such emotions lie in the deepest levels. Facial expression is human experience rendered immediately visible, without the intermediary of words.

Common sense originally meant *sensus communis*: the power to translate each sense into the other, without which no consciousness would be possible. In the tribal world, the eye listens, the ear sees and all the senses assist each other in concert, in a many-layered symphony of the senses, a cinematic flow which includes our 'five and country senses'.

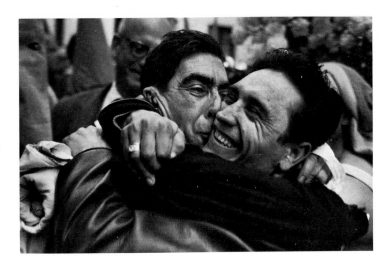

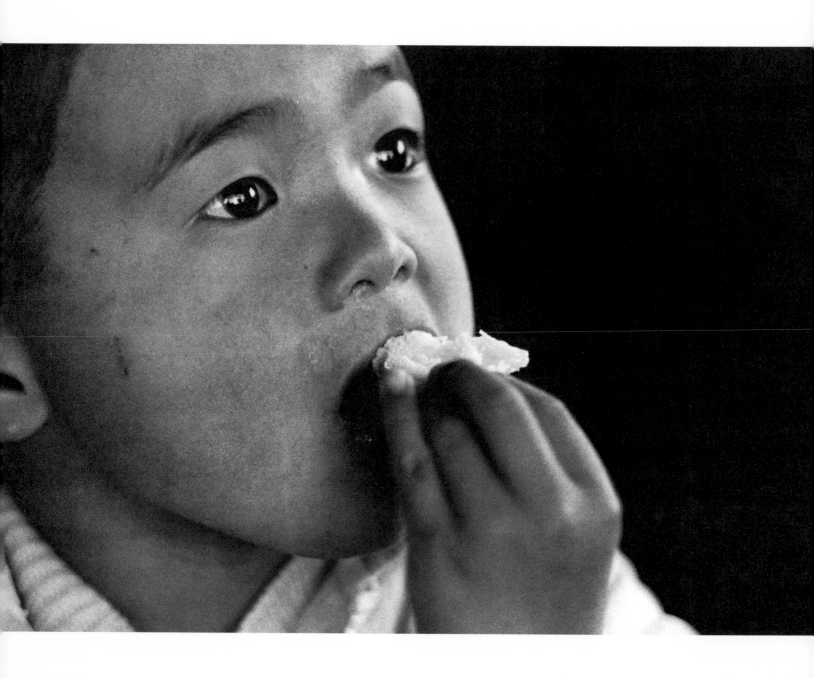

EDMUND LEACH

Taste and smell

Elsewhere in this book I have committed myself to the view that sensory experience is a totality and that if we describe the operations of the individual senses separately, one after another, we can only convey a very impoverished impression of what is going on. Now, under editorial coercion, I am embarked on doing precisely that for the two separated senses of taste and smell. For this artificial purpose I shall define taste as the discriminatory judgments which the individual makes on the basis of sensory inputs from the surface of the tongue, and smell as the corresponding discriminatory judgments that derive from sensory inputs from the nose. In practical terms such discriminations are not independent. Wine connoisseurs and professional tea-tasters are just as interested in the visual appearance and smell of the stuff as they are in how it tastes.

It is precisely in this area of discrimination, however, that taste and smell differ from the other three obvious sub-categories of sensation: sight, hearing, touch. If I utter the word *cat* there is a clear-cut beginning and a clear-cut end to the auditory signal; likewise the written word CAT has a visible beginning and a visible end; and if I stroke pussy in the dark I can feel where her nose begins and where her tail ends. But smells and tastes are not easily separable and segmentable in that sort of way. Without very special training it is hard to determine just where one taste or smell stimulus ends and another begins, and when tastes and smells overlie one another they merge to generate an atmosphere rather than the impression of a set of separable objects. The smell of spices in an oriental market is unmistakably evocative, but I doubt if even the most experienced inhabitants would be able to say on any particular occasion just which spices were present and which were not.

So we come to one immediate but negative conclusion. Because the 'messages' conveyed to the mind through the sense organs of taste and smell are *not* segmented, we can assert categorically that they are *not* structured 'like a language' even to the most elementary degree. A closely related point is that when we talk about taste and smell as isolates we are concerned only with the reception of sensory messages and not with their generation and transmission. In the case of spoken and written language, music, dance, and all the plastic arts of painting, sculpture, architecture, the actor or artist who is generating the 'message' has close control over the sensory images that are being transmitted so that, potentially at

The body desires us to eat, and has built us this succulent theatre of the mouth, all lit up with taste buds and papillae.
Paul Valéry

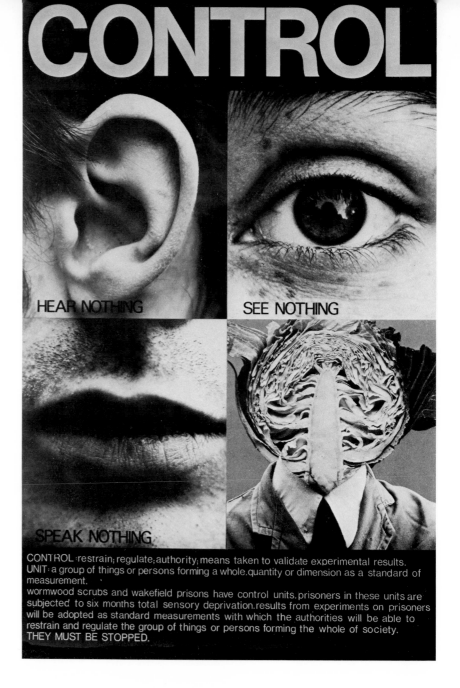

CONTROL

HEAR NOTHING

SEE NOTHING

SPEAK NOTHING

CONTROL restrain; regulate; authority; means taken to validate experimental results.
UNIT a group of things or persons forming a whole.quantity or dimension as a standard of measurement.
wormwood scrubs and wakefield prisons have control units.prisoners in these units are subjected to six months total sensory deprivation.results from experiments on prisoners will be adopted as standard measurements with which the authorities will be able to restrain and regulate the group of things or persons forming the whole of society.
THEY MUST BE STOPPED.

Denying sensory input, by depriving a prisoner of one or more of the senses, is a method of control used in prisons. A 'Radical Alternatives' poster protests against this way of reducing a human being to a mental cabbage.

least, there should be some sort of controlled relationship between the message that is sent out and the message that is received. Even in the case of speech this relationship is seldom a matter of one-to-one identity, and in the other creative arts it is very difficult to discover how far the message that was received corresponds to the intended message that was sent. My point here, though, is that with taste and smell even the possibility of such correspondence is remote.

Under emotional stimuli of various kinds – intense physical exertion, sex, excretion and so on – the human body emits strong odours which are characteristic both of the situation and of the individual concerned. But the individual who emits these odours does not monitor their emission and cannot control their production. We can, of course, in a ham-fisted way, override the operation of our personal olfactory processes either by frequent washing and the use of deodorants or by saturating the environment with some alternative smell. It is fairly obvious that smell has strong (unconscious as well as conscious) sexual connotations, and the cunning arts of perfume concoction have a history which goes back for millennia; but, like the closely related business of prescribing aphrodisiacs, this is a game which is more profitable to the producer than to the consumer. Despite all the contrary assertion of the advertising industry the response of either males or females to the smells emitted by members of either their own or the opposite sex is in the highest degree unpredictable and idiosyncratic.

There are also some striking differences at a cross-cultural level. Under the pressure of the advertisers contemporary North Americans have learnt to distinguish commercially produced 'perfumes', which are widely tolerated or even approved, from natural body odours which are universally condemned; in general, they now tend to associate cleanliness with a bland absence of distinctive smell. Any food market which generated a strong smell of any kind would immediately be rated as insanitary. By contrast, the whole Arab world of the Middle East has a long established convention that smell should be valued for its own sake. Not only are market-places rich in the odour of spices and incense but body smells are admitted as signs of personal identity.

By comparison with many other animals and even insects, our human sensitivity to smell appears very rudimentary, though it is difficult to know just how far this is due to inhibition or simple lack of capacity. It is striking that the smell which seems to evoke the most powerful reaction in human beings everywhere is the fetid stench of a rotting corpse. At a private level smell has intimate associations with excretion and with sex; at a public level it has a very direct association with death. On both accounts it is an area of sensation which is heavily subject to taboo. We react to smells all the time, but we do not talk about them very much, and, to judge by the relative paucity of information on the subject which appears in ethnographic monographs, this reticence must be universal.

We are less inhibited with regard to taste, but the categories of distinction are usually very vague. Our English terms 'sweet', 'sour', 'hot', 'cold', 'sharp', 'bitter', 'bland', 'mild', 'rich' and so on have their counterparts in other languages, though seldom with the same spread of meaning. In the contemporary West, equipped as we are with refrigerators and food preservatives, we tend to avoid food which has gone rotten and which on that account carries the smell-associations of death. In technologically less sophisticated cultures, especially in the tropics, a great deal of food, especially meat food, is 'bad' in the sense of 'rotten', but the associated smells and tastes tend to be masked by the intensive use of spices, especially 'hot' spices of the pepper-chili type. Notice, however, that even in the West, where 'bad' food is usually condemned as uneatable, some of the most prestigious delicacies (e.g. Stilton cheese) carry just that fetid stench of death which is otherwise avoided.

Clearly, it is the associations with death and sex which bring smells within the ambit of religious taboo. Equally clearly it is the involvement of oral, anal, and genital responses in the processes of infantile socialization together with the taboos surrounding the adult intimacies of sexual intercourse which bring taste into the same ambit, at least at the periphery. In all parts of the world myth and poetry and unconventional speech tend to treat eating and sexual intercourse as metaphorical equivalents: between lovers, the declaration 'I could eat you' does not suggest the prospect of cannibalism.

But smell can also serve as a metaphor for taste, and, in religious contexts where metaphysical beings are supposed to share in the commensality of a human congregation, this can be useful:

> And he shall take of it his handful, of the flour of the meat offering, and of the oil thereof, and all the frankincense which is upon the meat offering, and shall burn it upon the altar for a sweet savour . . . unto the Lord. (Leviticus 6:15)

What smell is to a man is taste to a God!

I remarked just now that smell creates a sense of a pervading atmosphere rather than of separable things, and the religious use of smells illustrates this point. Ritual proceedings must be marked off from the normal events of everyday life both in space and in time. Thus it is not sufficient that the proceedings take place in a specially allocated building such as a church; the specifically sacred nature of the occasion must be marked in some additional way – very commonly by means of music and other kinds of noise. But the special sanctity of ritual space may also be indicated by smell – the burning of incense. By convention, the smell of incense is rated as sweet and pleasant; whether it is 'really' all that different from the fetid smell of death is a point which only chemists and physiologists could decide. But in any case death, which is 'bitter' when it is located in the secular world of normality, is already 'sweet' by the time it has been removed to the sacred world of abnormality. The expression 'the odour of sanctity' was traditionally applied to the supposedly sweet smell of the corpse of a dead saint.

The general point that I am hinting at here is that in the whole field of taste and smell, precisely because it is very difficult to discriminate any objective boundaries, all judgments about good/bad or pleasant/unpleasant are wholly arbitrary. The root of our interest in smell and taste is essentially animal, hominid rather than human, and the biological focus is very narrow – sex, dead meat, and the body odours incorporated in excreta cover pretty well the whole of it. Taboo tends to inhibit our consciousness of these obsessions, but the underlying interest comes to the surface again in our preferred alternatives. The smell of human sexual secretions is 'dirty',

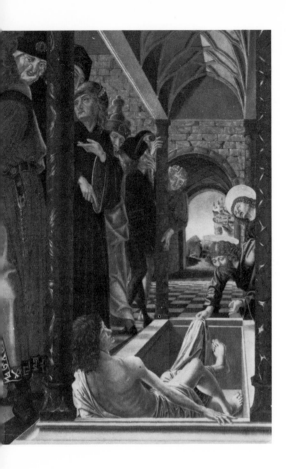

Michael Pacher, *The Raising of Lazarus*, from the St Wolfgang altarpiece, Salzkammergut.

but the legitimate substitute scents, the 'perfumes' of modern commerce, are compounded of the sexual secretions of animals and plants. Corpses are shunned but rotten cheese, rotten game and even rotten fish may be treated as delicacies – and the 'odour of sanctity' often has a marked resemblance to the odour of death.

So far, I have been implying that taste and smell are so closely allied as to be almost interchangeable, but the matter is not so simple. Whether I am conscious of the fact or not, every situation in which I find myself conveys a sense of atmosphere through the nose. In English, many verbal metaphors reflect this state of affairs: a noisy unpleasant quarrel is 'a stink'; 'a bad smell' implies suspicion of political corruption. But taste has in some respects just the opposite connotation: a 'man of taste' is a man of discrimination who generates his own atmosphere; 'bad taste' is not vicious or corrupt, it simply displays pretentiousness and lack of education. The point is that whereas we are bound to pick up continuous smell impressions of the atmosphere simply because we breathe, tasting with the tongue is an intentional act, a testing of a specially selected sample of experience. These are English language usages, but the background is more general. In the first place, the elaboration of food preparation as a culinary art has been a peculiarity of a small number of outstandingly affluent civilizations, and the appreciation of that art by tasting has been a specialization developed in the first place by members of the ruling elite of such societies. Secondly, however, it must be realized that tasting with the tongue relies in part on a sense of touch. When we taste something we do not simply discriminate sensations such as sweet and bitter, or flavours where such reactions are compounded with smell; we also make judgments about texture – the food is smooth or gritty, tough or tender, viscous or free-flowing, and so on. So, despite the point which I made right at the beginning about the absence of segmentation in the normal flow of our taste and smell sensations, it is still the case that, because taste is really a combination of a variety of different kinds of impression including smell and touch, we can use it to make very fine discriminations. Fox has described the taxonomic procedures of Pinatubo Negrito botanists in the following terms:

> Many times I have seen a Negrito who, when not being certain of the identification of a particular plant, will taste the fruit, smell the leaves, break and examine the stem, comment upon its habitat, and only after this pronounce whether he did or did not know the plant.

But that simply takes us back to where I started. It is misleading to suppose that we possess separable senses which we use one at a time. We possess multiple senses which are all operating simultaneously, and the impressions they convey to our consciousness are the outcome of a computation process in which all these simultaneous messages are combined with a feed-back derived from past experience and future expectation. The operations which we describe as smelling and tasting are no more than facets of a much more elaborate system of total sense impressions.

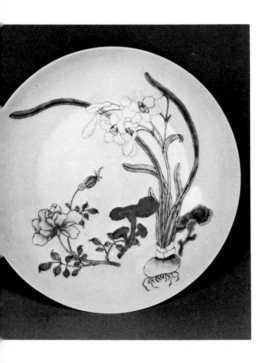

The flowery visual symbol of yin decorating this dish contains qualities to be transmitted to the food that is placed in the dish. The qualities are then absorbed by whoever eats the food. *Famille rose* porcelain, mid eighteenth century.

123

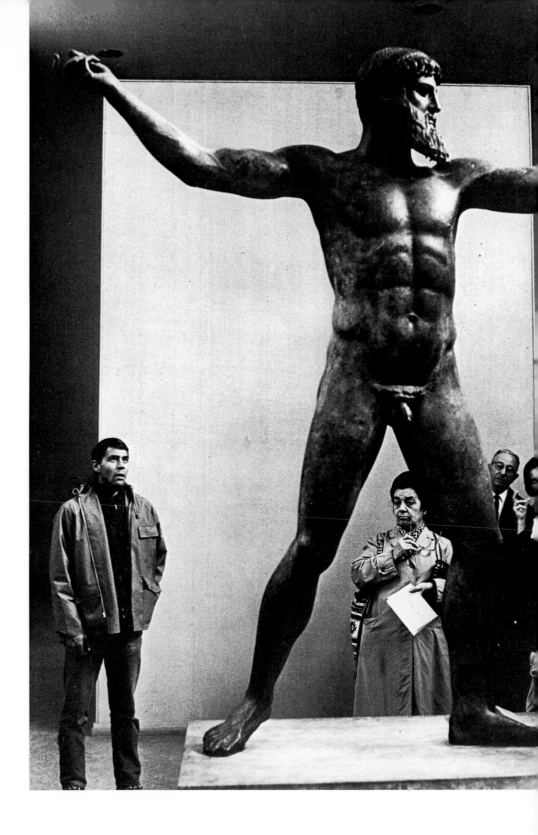

He who cannot see himself within the context of at least a 2,000-year expanse of history is all his life shackled to days and weeks.
Rainer Maria Rilke

EDWARD LUCIE-SMITH Sensibility and history

Edward Lucie-Smith is a poet and an art critic. His books include *The Well Wishers, British Poetry Since 1945*, and *Movements in Art Since 1945*. His two most recent books are a biography of Joan of Arc and *Arte Oggi*.

Western theories of art have once more begun to veer towards the notion (which probably has its roots in the early *Sturm und Drang* phase of the Romantic Movement) that what counts, in the spectator's reaction to the object, is the instinctive movement of feeling at the first moment of encounter. From this has sprung an increasing hostility to art criticism. The critic, it is felt, not only has no standing in the matter, but is actually less well rather than better equipped to achieve a full communion with the work of art. What obstructs him is what is generally called, rather scornfully, his 'tendency to intellectualize'. The pages which follow, though not intended as a defence of criticism, are intended to put forward the idea that we greatly oversimplify our approach to many works of art, and misunderstand the way in which they work on us.

Indeed, it is not too much to say that, by turning the 'leap of feeling' into a principle as mandatory as the 'leap of faith' became to the theologians of the late Middle Ages, we in fact coarsen our approach to many art works to the point where we miss nearly everything they have to offer us.

The two notions which must first be cleared out of the way are these: that the work of art functions in precisely the same way in every context; and that the modern artist in particular can revert, merely by an act of will, to the role which the shaman-artist played in relation to the primitive society that produced him. The first idea, erroneous as it is, is more or less a commonplace among art-lovers. It is bound up with the concept of the masterpiece, that is, of the work of art which, thanks to the power compacted within itself, oversteps all temporal and social boundaries, and achieves a universal meaning.

The second notion is chiefly professed by those who think of themselves as being in some way 'radical' in their approach to art and its problems, and is based on the kind of false primitivism which somehow holds that technology has returned us full circle, to the condition in which we began. The easiest means of disproving this theory is by reference to the universally accepted distinction between primitive and developed cultures. It is that primitive art, the product of a tribal matrix, shows no real dynamism. It cannot develop or transform itself because the culture which produces it is too rigid. Once the mould is cracked – as was the case when the tribes of Africa and Oceania came into collision with the West – a rapid degeneration

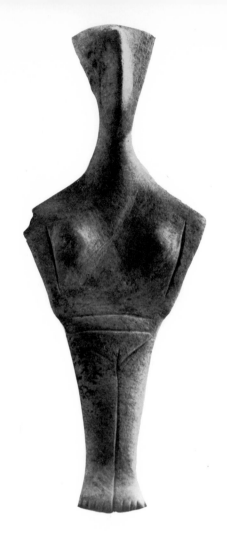

takes place. On the other hand, the great civilizations, those of India and China as well as our own, have shown a consistent though not inexhaustible power of self-transformation and therefore of self-renewal.

The huge array of works of primitive art filling so many major museums in England, Europe and the United States provides an excellent means of testing our reactions to the aesthetic experience. Until comparatively recently, it was hardly admitted that such objects were 'art' at all. Those who first collected them, and in many cases brought them to the institutions where they now repose, thought of them as being things of chiefly scientific interest, contributions to a rational study of the development of mankind. The arrangement of many leading ethnographical collections bears witness to the fact that this attitude still lingers, in however attenuated a form. The objects are presented not for their own sake, as Old Master paintings usually are, but as fragments of information about a particular culture or set of beliefs.

This attitude is not, however, borne out by our own reactions to these objects when we are confronted with them. Most present-day spectators feel a ready response to the smooth, precise forms of a Dan mask, or to the violent expressionism of certain tribal objects from New Guinea or the New Hebrides. It is certainly true that we have been taught by developments in our own culture to look at these things with fresh eyes. The borrowings from primitive art made by modern artists, from Picasso and Braque onwards, have enabled us to incorporate much into our own universe of feeling. In addition – and here is something which is perhaps more important – we have also witnessed, in the course of the past half-century, the rapid expansion of what André Malraux dubbed the *musée imaginaire*. In Malraux's terms, the *musée imaginaire* is the whole vast spectrum of works of art which are available, even if only in reproduction, to the contemporary spectator. Modern developments in transportation, technological advances in both printing and photography, have immensely increased the number of paintings, sculptures and art-objects which each of us may claim to have seen, in comparison with the members of previous generations.

The result of this familiarity with a huge and heterogeneous mass of material has not, as Malraux points out, been entirely beneficial. In the first place there is the risk that people will become so glutted with images that few, even the most powerful, will make any impression on them. Secondly, and this is perhaps more serious, the multiplicity of objects, representing a multiplicity of civilizations and tribal cultures, which now form part of our consciousness, has removed the last remaining pretence of cultural unity. We are now the heirs, directly or indirectly, not of one culture but of many.

The spectator who walks into an ethnographical museum probably comes equipped with at least a hazy general notion of what he is going to see, and he may depart, thanks to the efforts of an intelligent curator, with a much clearer idea of the social and religious background of the objects on view than he had when he went in.

Cycladic idol from Pharos, c. 2000 BC.

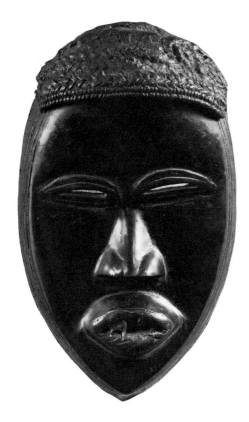

But it is ridiculous to suppose that even the most skilful piece of museum display can make him experience the things he sees as they were designed in the first place to be experienced by the men who made them. For one thing, many objects formed an integral part of rituals which were performed only at special seasons or in special circumstances, perhaps in secrecy; often the most important details of these are completely lost to us, and even the expert is forced to resort to conjecture to fill the gaps in his laboriously acquired knowledge.

The visitor therefore has to try to make a bridge to what he is looking at out of his own resources, which consist of a mixture of physical perception, past experience and fantasy. Perhaps it will be useful to try and define these three terms a little more closely. By physical perception I mean the information the senses give us. With the visual arts we depend chiefly on the sense of sight, particularly in museums, where we are not allowed to touch the objects. By experience, I mean what we have stored in our memories, the echoes and re-echoes of other things seen which the object we are looking at produces. A piece of African sculpture may perhaps remind us of the way a certain plant tends to grow, and of our associations with that particular plant –

Wooden dance mask of the Dan tribes on the Ivory Coast, 20th century.

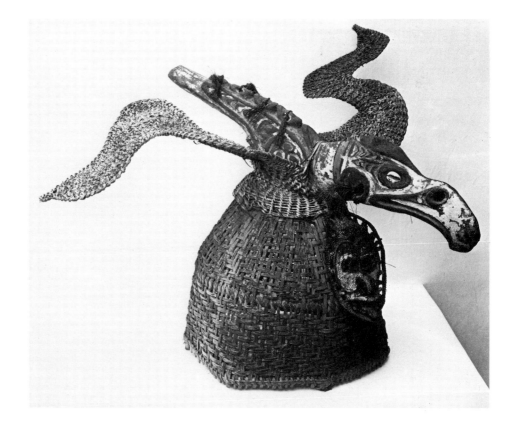

Basketry mask from the Sepik River area of New Guinea.

associations which may well be irrelevant to other people but which are genuinely moving to us. This takes me to the border of what I have called 'fantasy'. Fantasy is something which pre-exists in our own psyche, but which is aroused or triggered off by the presence of the work of art. Through fantasy it is possible for an object of whose true history and origins we are virtually ignorant to arouse a powerful emotional response.

Strangely enough, some of the most ardent advocates of the 'leap of feeling' are suspicious of fantasy and of all that the concept implies. For one thing, giving fantasy a prime and legitimate place seems to remove the division between the work of art and the natural object: it puts a piece of sculpture which has come down to us from some little-known ancient civilization upon much the same footing as some curiously shaped fragment of rock, shaped by wind and weather alone without human intervention.

The common-sense objection that we *know* the sculpture to be not only ancient but shaped by the hand of man, and therefore feel differently about it and react in a different way, convicts us of an impurity of attitude, a refusal to let what we see act upon us as directly as it ought. 'Suppose the thing turned out to be a modern fake,' the sceptic jeers; 'wouldn't you feel differently about it then?' The answer is that of course one would, and that this is another example of the way foreknowledge inevitably influences aesthetic response, neither more nor less striking than the contrary example I have already given. My contention would be that it is inevitably impossible to divorce what we feel from what we know, with the proviso that it is not by any means mandatory to know everything about the work of art in order to enjoy it. This, too, is a matter of common sense.

Given the ambiguity of the contemporary situation, how can we most profitably approach the work of art? There is, of course, no magic formula which will bring pictures and sculptures alive to those who have hitherto been indifferent to them, just as there is no way of teaching the tone-deaf listener to enjoy Beethoven. Some things, however, are bound to help. The first is the decision to concentrate simply on what is there. We often think we have 'seen' a work of art simply because we have been for a few seconds in its presence. When the *Mona Lisa* was sent to America, tens of thousands of people filed past the spot where it hung – but how many of them actually saw it in any meaningful sense? If we have truly seen something, we ought to be able, afterwards, to give a reasonably accurate description of it, and it is quite a useful exercise for the novice museum-visitor to write down a brief account of what he has seen when he gets home.

At the same time, we must be careful that the eye doesn't fatigue itself. If we glare at a single work for a long period, we gradually feel its meaning draining away, rather than increasing. And this is not surprising, since the natural way to look at things is to scan them, to observe them from different angles and distances. This varied way of perceiving things through the sense of sight is one of the things which the camera cannot give us.

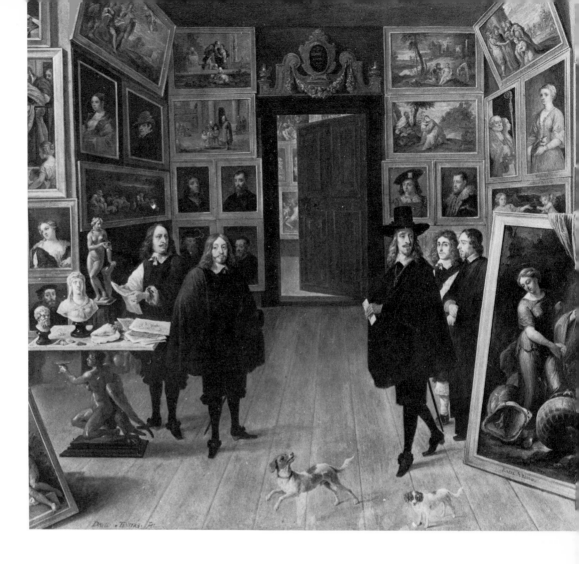

Detail of painting by David Teniers the younger,
Gallery of the Archduke Leopold at Brussels.

Most important of all, perhaps, is the effort to be certain that we truly saw what was truly there: 'Is that how it was, or is that how it was supposed to be?' Too often, when we look at a very celebrated work of art, we have in our heads a recollection of how other men have looked at it and described it. We must always ask if their reactions are valid for ourselves. If there is a difference, we must ask why that difference exists.

So far, for the sake of clarity of argument, I have mostly been dealing with works of art which fall into a category which is obviously very far removed from ourselves – the products of a totally different environment. But what about the works which spring from our own tradition – the legacy of the long development of Western civilization? We would, I think, like to feel closer to these than in fact we are. When we survey some of the universally accepted key works of the Western medieval and

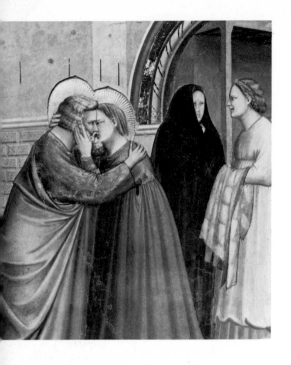

post-medieval tradition, we are, if we are honest, struck by the distance which now separates the circumstances in which they were produced from those in which we now live.

For one thing, many of the most famous are the product of the Christian religion, and the Christian myth is now under siege in a way which must inevitably affect our response to what we are looking at. The moving quality of Michelangelo's *Pietà* in St Peter's, or of Giotto's frescoes in Padua, is inextricably bound up with their relationship to a faith which many people no longer profess, or which they profess in so lukewarm a way that the sacred story, though it remains familiar, has lost most of its impact.

I can perhaps demonstrate some of the implications of this change by considering a famous series of paintings by Poussin, and its possible impact on a modern audience. The series is the set of *Seven Sacraments* now on loan to the National Gallery of Scotland. The paintings are by any standards austere and difficult to approach. The symbolism reflects, if not Jansenism itself, then the most rigorous and puritan aspect of seventeenth-century French Catholicism. Poussin distances familiar New Testament scenes, not only by the stiff and rigid way in which he paints his figures, but by putting them into classical dress and into a classical setting. As Mary Magdalen washes his feet, Jesus reclines on a Roman banqueting couch. Yet, even for the uninstructed spectator, the paintings have an immediate effect, which springs not from their subject-matter but from the splendid rhythm of the forms – the pictorial equivalent of a Bach cantata.

It is perhaps not too much to suppose that the contemporary spectator sees Poussin's *Seven Sacraments* not only in a different, but also in a diametrically opposite, manner from that in which they would have been seen by the audience for whom the artist originally worked. That is, the contemporary spectator grasps the formal qualities of the pictures with little difficulty, indeed instinctively, but has to make a conscious effort to apprehend the subject-matter. But this latter, for all the aloofness of its presentation, would of course have had an immediate impact in the seventeenth century.

All this leads me to a conclusion totally contrary to the one usually accepted today. It seems to me that the powers of generalization and conceptualization with which we have been endowed by the progress of Western thought (and also of Western technology) during the past two hundred and fifty years actually make it easier to respond to the work of art because they teach us to discard what is in fact inessential. If one looks back at the development, not of art itself, but of art criticism, one is startled to discover how much more delicate and precise its techniques of analysis, and even of description, have become. Diderot, who has some claims to be the first art critic in the modern sense of the term, dissatisfies us now because his language seems not to fit his purpose. When a painting moves him by its emotional strength, he is too often forced to attribute what he feels merely to its subject-matter, because he has evolved no method of describing a direct confrontation with

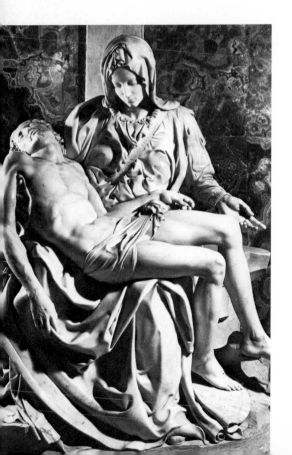

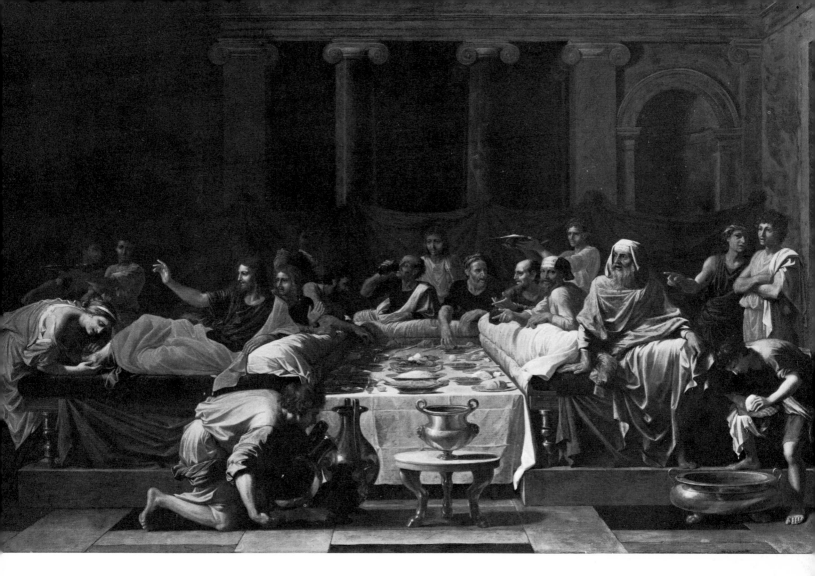

Above: Nicolas Poussin, *The Sacrament of Penance*, 1644–48.

Opposite, above: Anna and Joachim – detail of Giotto's fresco *Meeting at the Golden Gate* in the Scrovegni Chapel, Padua; 14th century.

Opposite, below: Michelangelo's *Pietà*, 1499, in St Peter's, Rome.

the work of art. Similarly, Browning's much-admired monologues about painters and painting turn out to be almost entirely anecdotal – the only way in which the poet can approach what Andrea del Sarto produced is through the stories Vasari tells us about the artist's matrimonial difficulties.

The classical strain in modern art, the passion for ordering visual sensations into forms which calm the spirit by their own tranquil stability, is matched by our interest in a very different kind of art which nakedly and sometimes frenziedly reveals the personality of the artist. The man who, in the first half of the twentieth century, most successfully combined these two aspects was undoubtedly Picasso. The relationship between the two halves of his artistic personality is often paradoxical. The *Demoiselles d'Avignon*, which is the starting-point of Cubism, is also a fierce assault

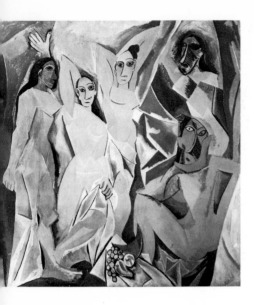

Picasso, *Les Demoiselles d'Avignon.*

Van Gogh, *Self-Portrait with a Bandaged Ear.*

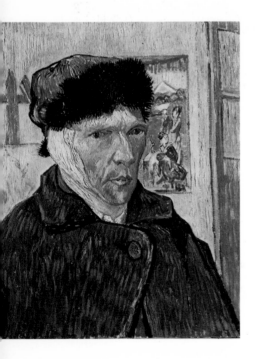

on everything which people thought beautiful at the time it was painted. Picasso's treatment of the theme of the Minotaur gives us horrifying yet curiously exhilarating views of creative anger and anguish.

Picasso, however, was by no means the first artist to use his art as a means of asserting the rights of the ego. Western artists had long fostered within themselves an awareness of the self, as we can see from numerous self-portraits dating from the fifteenth century onwards. But now the artist becomes a consciously alienated individual – triumphant yet abject, exalted yet despairing. We already catch more than a glimpse of this in early Romantics such as Fuseli, and by Van Gogh's day the pattern was set. Van Gogh's rejection by an unfeeling bourgeois public, his madness and suicide, are by this time clichés so thoroughly established in our minds that we are in danger of forgetting what the pictures have to say. Compare, for instance, the great late self-portrait by Rembrandt with Van Gogh's *Self-Portrait with a Bandaged Ear*. Rembrandt was, around 1663 when he painted this picture, a failure in the material sense. His health was also deteriorating. He confronts these facts and puts them down unsparingly. But his picture has none of the savagery of Van Gogh's, none of the absolute immediacy of personal pain, physical and spiritual. And ever since Van Gogh's day artists have continued to believe in the legitimacy of their right to unleash the forces they feel boiling within themselves, to immerse us in a maelstrom where we may sink or swim as we please. This maelstrom is the metaphor which lies behind the frenzied calligraphy of Jackson Pollock.

Knowledge of the *musée imaginaire* brings home to us the fact that all subjects are legitimate in art. But emphasis on the alienated status of the artist has tended to corrupt our approach to the visual arts by tempting us to transfer our attention from the object to its creator. In the end, as certain anonymous works ought to teach us, it is the object which counts. The tremendous calm of Old Kingdom portraits from Ancient Egypt is an abstract quality which nevertheless exists objectively, in the stone of the statue itself. It does not matter that we do not know who made these things, nor what was in his mind at the time he made them. Another test-case, where the author at least is known but the intention is still veiled, is Rembrandt's *The Flayed Ox*. Why is this representation of a carcass so moving? It is superficial to see in it simply an allegory of man's own mortality; it is equally superficial to praise it only for the painter's mastery of his craft, his ability to make us say 'how beautiful' to what we might not find beautiful in real life. When we look at it we know it enhances our sense of being, enlarges our idea of what a man can be. We do not experience so great an enlargement when we look at one of Soutine's versions of the same subject. The reason is, perhaps, that we feel the portrayal is less objective. The emotion which has been added adventitiously by the artist diminishes rather than enhances our own responses.

In his book, *A Voice from the Chorus*, which consists chiefly of notes made during his six years in a Soviet forced labour camp, Andrey Sinyavsky has a passage on museums:

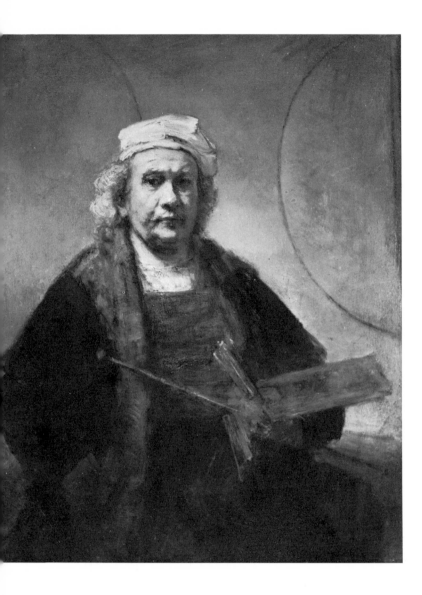

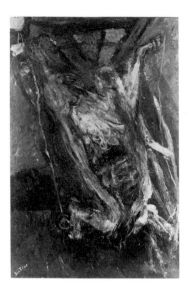

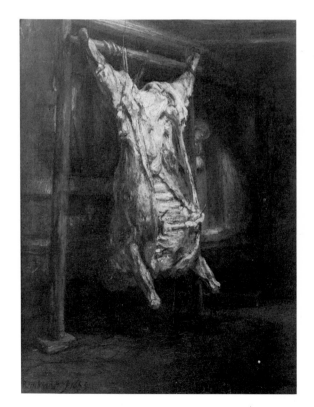

Rembrandt, *Self-Portrait*, c.1663.

Lower right: Rembrandt, *Flayed Ox*; *top right:*
Chaim Soutine's version of the same subject.

Works of art, unlike books, provide an environment in which you can live – they surround you like the trees in a forest and gradually permeate your being in the same way as any other habitat. Forests and museums – these are what I should like to go to; they are somehow intertwined in my memory, and are what I miss most.

It seems to me that these sentences come somewhere near the heart of the matter. The emotion we feel in the presence of a work of art is not the same emotion we would feel in the presence of the thing depicted (granted always that the painting or sculpture concerned is figurative and not abstract). In fact, what we experience is a feeling about the presence of feeling, an emotion which is also an analysis. To put it another way, the work of art is itself neutral; it acts as a catalyst, energizes emotions which already existed within us, and which now combine, like chemicals, in new ways. Yet a third way of looking at it is to say that visual art – painting and sculpture – is an important bridge between man and his environment, the enemy of alienation, not the expression of it. This is because in this field we see how substance becomes idea, and vice versa. Michelangelo's *Pietà* in St Peter's does not cease to be stone because of the form the artist has given it. And indeed it is Michelangelo himself, in one of his sonnets, who speaks of the form lying already within the rock, and waiting to be freed by the sculptor's chisel. Possibility is the great gift made to us by works of art. Apparently inanimate, they challenge us by changing as we look at them, and every time we look.

Opposite: Hopewell Cult hand of sheet metal, found buried with an American Indian in Ohio; dated to 300 BC–AD 500.

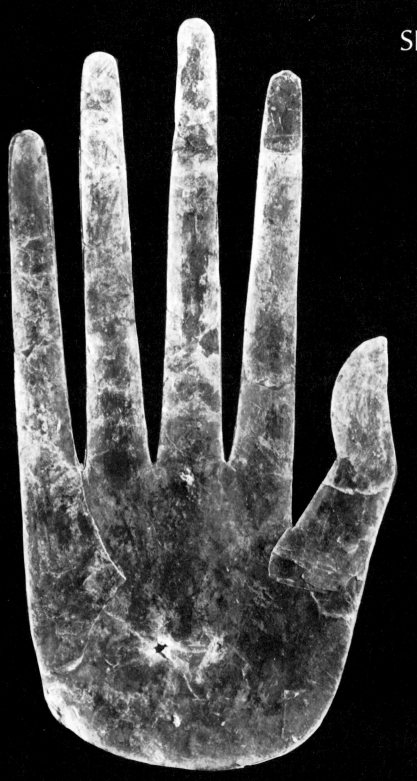

SENSORY ENRICHMENT: artists lead the way

The task of all deep religions — especially Buddhism — or of really good therapy, is the satori, the great awakening, the coming to one's senses, waking up from one's dream ... When we come to our senses, we start to see, to feel, to experience.

Fritz Perls

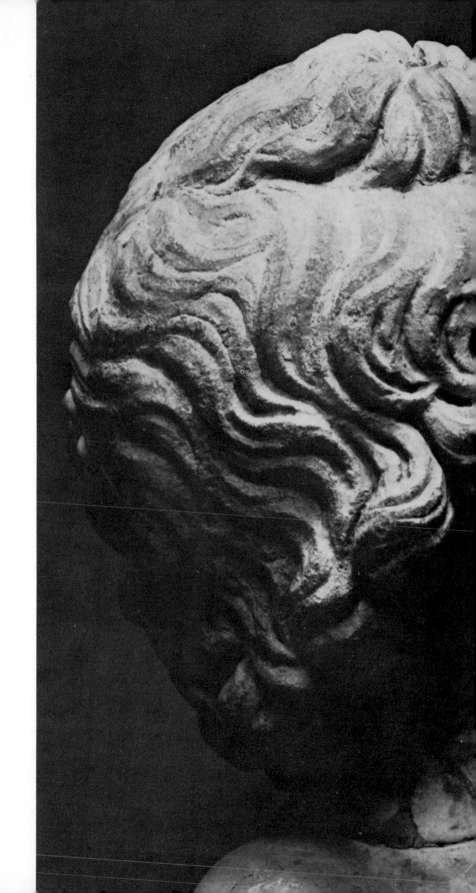

Statue of Cupid and Psyche (detail).

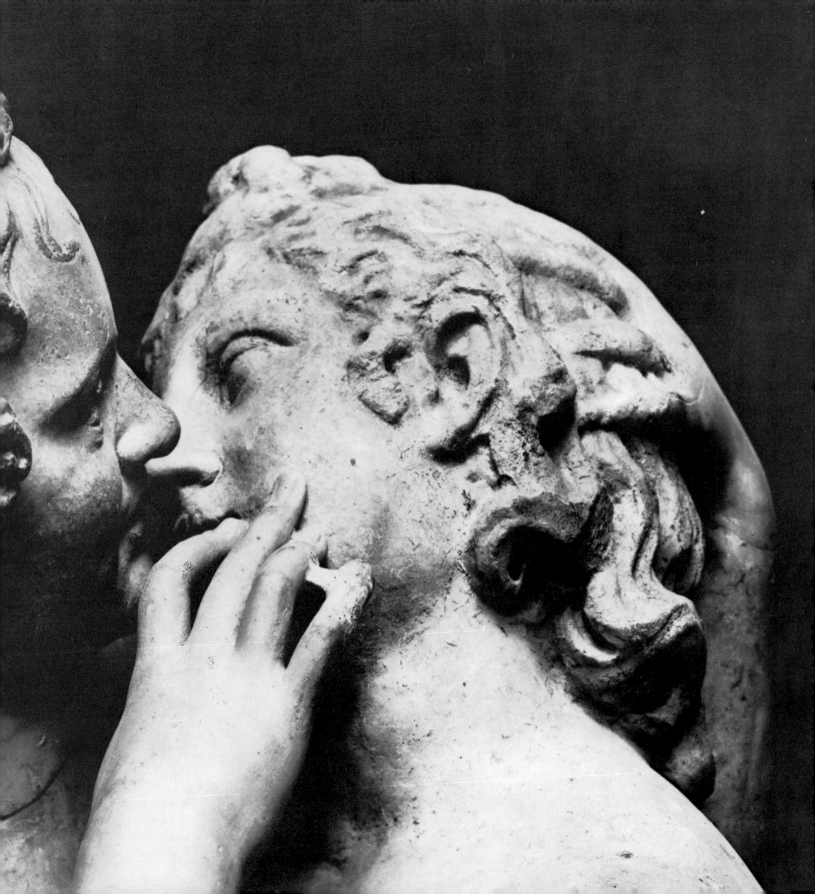

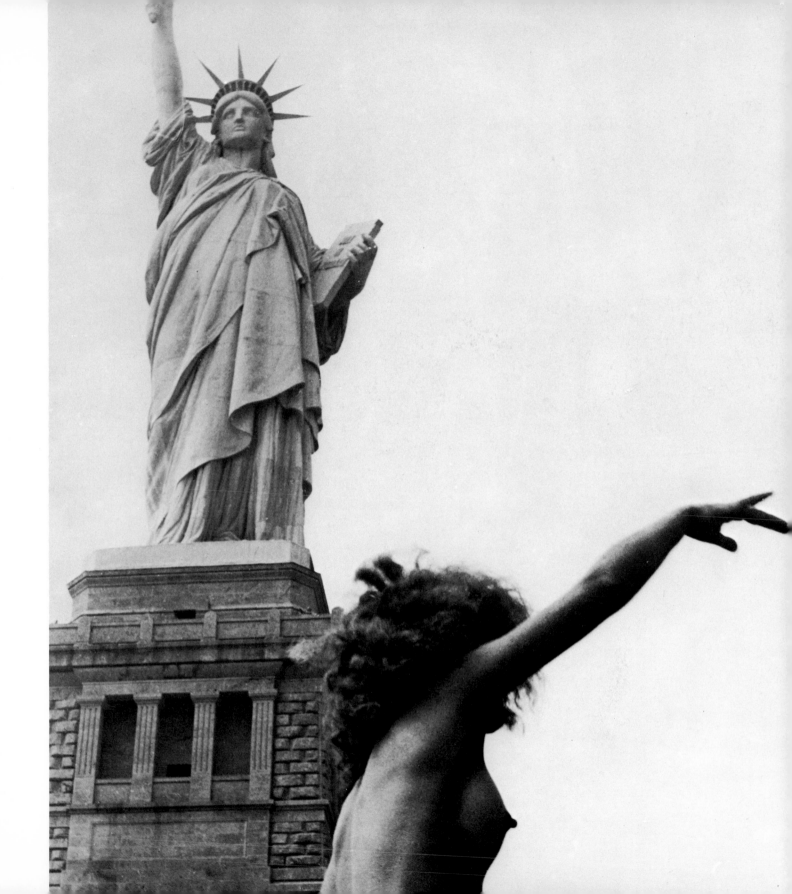

CAROLINE TISDALL

Caroline Tisdall is an art critic for the *Guardian* newspaper, in London. She also lectures in twentieth-century art history at the University of Reading and has mounted several major art exhibitions in Europe and America.

Every human being is an artist

The traditional role of art has been the cultivation and nurturing of the senses. In the greatest art of all times and places this has never been an end in itself, however: the senses give access to transcendental or spiritual experience, bringing about a synthesis of physical and spiritual awareness. Once this synthesizing potential is lost in a culture, the society itself begins to disintegrate.

In the sixties, many artists became aware that they were functioning within just such a disintegrating society. In the sick and divided body of modern society, art and the artist had become an almost expendable extremity of nebulous function. The poorer modern man becomes in both spiritual and sensual experience, the more marginal becomes the role of the artist. The synthesizing potential is lost.

Ideally, what art has to offer is the experience of the world through the whole spectrum of human perception: intuition, reason, emotion and sensation. The creation of a work of art involves all of these. A work that springs simply from instinct is as incomplete as one that is based only on analysis. Yet the artist as a specialist in modern society operates within the divided spectrum established by classic Western philosophy in which these areas are separated. The various senses, too, are categorized and read as quite clearly distinguishable, even to the extent that they are allocated different ranks in a hierarchy. Aristotle could claim that the visual sense, the painter's realm, was the only trustworthy sense since it was closest to the analytical function.

The ultimate irony is, of course, that in a society based on the notion of specialists in every field, the artist's audience, if he has one at all, is a passive audience. The active transmission of sensual and spiritual experience becomes all the more improbable. Art, if it is perceived, is taken as a tolerable eccentricity, a relaxing entertainment (Matisse's armchair), or as a specialist language to be analysed by those who know the language. Marx defined the forming of the five senses as the labour of the entire history of the world down to the present, yet according to his gauge, it is the very people who deal above all with the senses who are most alienated from their product in modern society.

The development of modernism – the mainstream of twentieth-century art – exemplifies this alienation. The mainstream from Cubism on has been a hermetic succession of changing styles. Each added something to the vocabulary of a

Yayoi Kusama, *'Naked Event' at Statue of Liberty*, 1968.

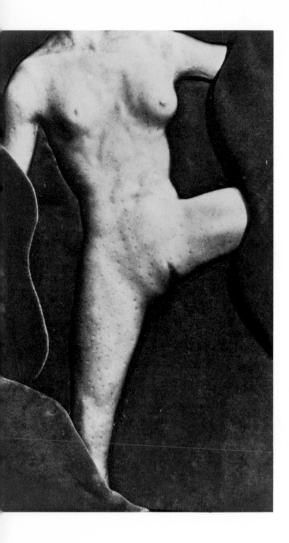

Marcel Duchamp, *Etant Donnés le Gaz d'Eclairage et la Chute d'Eau,* 1948–49.

specialist language, but accepted its limitations. Participation in the language became dependent on knowledge of its successive stages. As art became more self-referential, the result was a steadily increasing formalism and a correspondingly diminishing content, reaching a logical extreme of sensual and spiritual poverty in the American minimalism of the mid-sixties, where nothing was left but the brute materialism of the basic matter-of-fact object; everything else had been whittled away.

It is not surprising that the wider human awareness of recent years should have brought a reaction, based not simply on the realization of the sensual poverty of formalist art or the limitations of Clement Greenberg's 'aesthetic surprise'. Art itself as a restricted specialization divorced from all other areas of life was called into question. There were moves to extend the boundaries of art, to make it more relevant to contemporary experience, and to involve a wider public in a less passive way. Above all, the limitation of creativity to a specialist group called artists, custodians of the senses, was questioned by artists themselves. The radical position shifted from Robert Rauschenberg's search for an art that could 'bridge the gap between art and life' to Joseph Beuys' 'Every human being is an artist.'

But the movements that have contributed to this change of attitude – happenings, participation art, the Fluxus movement, performance and action art, land and body art – did not happen out of the blue. Historically they can be traced back through a succession of movements that have challenged the restrictions of the mainstream throughout the century. A seminal influence on the art of the sixties was, for instance, the Dada movement of the First World War: an outraged response to the mechanistic positivism and bourgeois materialism that had brought about that international holocaust. To counter destructive rational logic, the Dadaists proposed irrationality, instinct and the sensual release that was taken up and developed by the Surrealists with their emphasis on the liberating influence of the unleashed unconscious.

But these earlier movements laid a nostalgic emphasis on total irrationality and instinct that does not match the contemporary need for balance. To rely entirely on instinct and intuition, as some members of the Fluxus movement did, would now be as self-defeating and illusory as a Luddite return to the fields. The most significant moves towards a wider concept of art have been those which once established a balance between the senses and the thinking fields of perception and awareness. Here the paradoxical influence of Marcel Duchamp has remained amazingly fruitful. Duchamp has been many things to many artists: the logical anti-logician who upset the hierarchy of art by introducing the 'ready-made' (found object) as a work of art: the inventor of the truly mechanistic love-act, *The Bride Stripped Bare by her Bachelors, Even;* the great alchemist, and the sensualist whose last great work, revealed after his death, was a lyrical homage to erotic earthly love and its spiritual attributes. Duchamp was further relevant because he challenged the equation of art with the media of painting and sculpture. He rejected painting over fifty years ago as

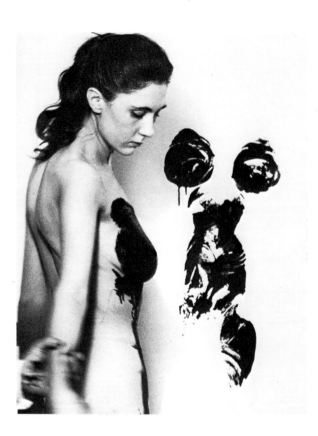

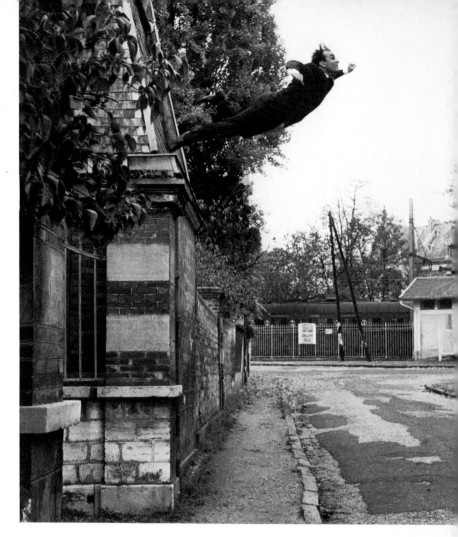

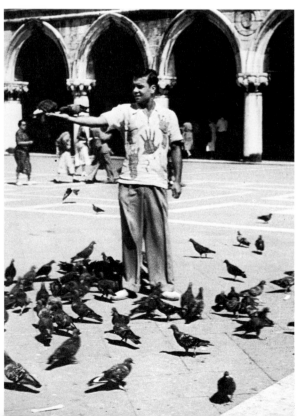

Yves Klein's *Leap Into the Void*, 1962.

Top left: nude girl used by Yves Klein as a 'living brush' in one of his *Anthropométries. Left:* Yves Klein wearing a shirt of his own design.

To project my mark outside myself – but I did it! My hands and feet impregnated with colour, I found myself confronting everything that was psychological in me. I had proof that I had five senses, that I knew how to get myself to function! And then I lost my childhood.
Yves Klein

141

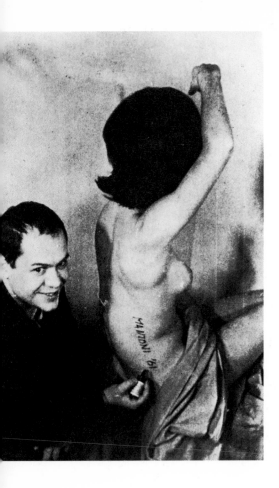

being simply 'retinal' – directed towards one sense – and 'olfactory' – laden with the smell of turps. He wanted an art that appealed to the mind as well and brought in elements of science, alchemy and mysticism. In terms of the emphasis laid on the senses in recent art, Duchamp's influence was characteristically paradoxical. On the one hand his example in challenging the limitations of art was expanded by those exploring new means as described later in this chapter. But he also laid the grounds for the analytical approach of the drier kind of conceptual art and endless theorizing.

Towards the end of the fifties, two more significant figures in the search for an expanded and totalized art emerged: the French artist Yves Klein and the Italian Piero Manzoni. They presented a fascinating balance to the more materialist development in the art of those years: Pop. Klein's programme was extravagantly sensual, and mystical to boot. He proposed the Blue Revolution: the transformation of sensibility through perception of the infinite, time and space opened up by his 'International Klein Blue' (IKB), and was influenced by the writings of Bachelard. Painting with fire and rain as well as his use of gold reinforced the ritualistic and alchemical tone of his activities, the most spectacular of which was his (unsuccessful) attempt to merge with space in unaided flights. Klein used nudes as 'living brushes' in his *Anthropométries*: canvases stained with the blue traces of their bodies and movements. Manzoni took a more radical step towards art as life. He created the 'Base for Living Sculpture' on to which anyone could step, and he signed nude bodies as 'living works of art', carrying Duchamp's idea of the 'ready-made' into warm flesh and proposing that art is a state of being. In the same way, everything that is processed by the artist, including his breath, blood and shit, was designated art. Apart from challenging once more the hierarchy of the art object, that also brought him into the area of taboo in Western society: the reversibility of the creative act and the act of defecation.

The exploration and demonstration of areas of bodily taboo has continued to play its part in art since then. It was very much part and parcel of the international Fluxus movement in Europe, America and Japan in the early sixties. Sexual morality was ridiculed in many uninhibited performances with women artists like Carolee Schleeman at last well to the fore. A series of Fluxus festivals generated the kind of communal and joyful excitement that was later to become characteristic of pop festivals, and one of the most endearing figures in these was the American artist Charlotte Moorman, stripped to the waist and playing the cello, her breasts concealed by miniature television sets as a wry comment on a spectator society that takes its pleasures well-processed by the media. Such events also laid the ground for a questioning of a male-dominated culture which promotes recognizably masculine values. Interest in other cultures has provided other models: the emphasis on the feminine nature of creativity in the art of India and the fusion of the two in Tantra played their part in balancing the suppression of the feminine side in Western culture. Interestingly enough, since male artists have suffered almost as much as

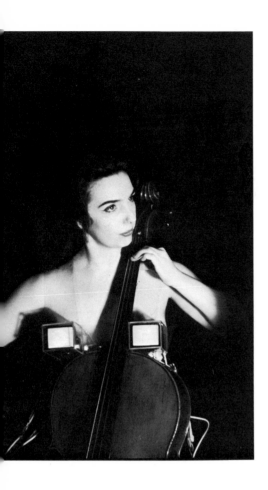

Charlotte Moorman, *TV Bra for Living Sculpture,*
1969.

Vettor Pisani, *L'eroe da camera, tutte le parole dal
silenzio di Duchamp al rumore di Beuys,* 1973.

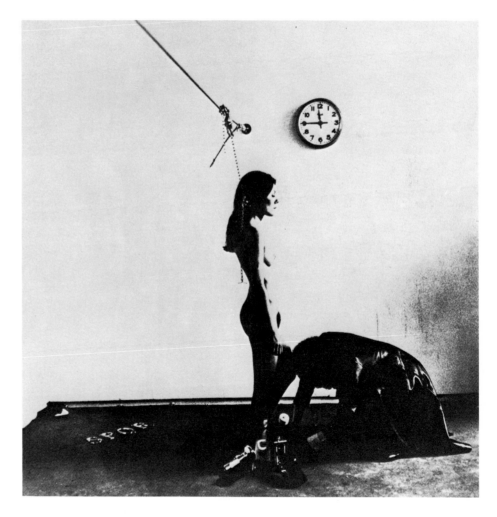

143

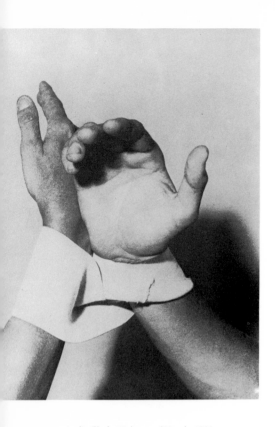

Lydia Clark, *Dialogue of Hands*, 1966

Meret Oppenheim, *Objet (Le Déjeuner en Fourrure)*, 1936.

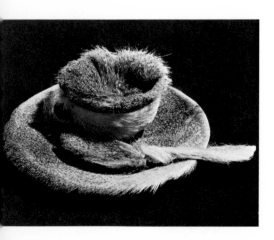

women through this particular taboo, a number of male artists have themselves proposed a more relaxed, ambiguous or androgynous position. Here again, Duchamp set a precedent through his alter ego: Rrose Sélavy – the fusion of the two sides of human nature in *Eros c'est la vie, Aimer tes héros* in a series of puns on life, love and sexual interchangeability or fusion. Some of the more flamboyant dressing-up activities of recent years, like those of the Swiss artist Urs Lüthi, have come close to the popular art of drag, and do little more than simply place that in an art context. The Italian artists Luigi Ontani and Vettor Pisani have taken it a step further, Ontani by referring back to the androgynous presence in the art of the past, and Pisani by complicating the constellation through direct reference to Duchamp and his own sister. The most mischievous exponent of the art of sexual liberation is still the silver screen persona of Andy Warhol: 'I think I'm missing some responsibility chemicals and some reproductive chemicals.'

A much more savage way of drawing attention to contemporary man's divided state has been developed by the most extreme exponents of alienation. The Austrian artists Hermann Nitsch, Günther Brus and Arnulf Rainer produced performances and tableaux in the sixties that were too strong a medicine for Vienna. They were expelled and have since settled in Berlin. The Viennese Orgien Misterien Theatre was accepted as a calculated measuring tool for the man-made phenomena of recorded time and constructed space. In England, Stuart Brisley has delved into the blacker side of a world of physical cruelty in a series of performances over the last ten years, ranging from totally white antiseptic eating situations to days spent immersed in a black bath of stinking offal. Nothing could be further from the traditional image of the gentle artist as guardian of the senses in a smiling society.

Other artists have devised more therapeutic art forms designed to remedy such extremes of alienation. The early exponents of participation art, particularly the Brazilian artists Lydia Clark and Helio Oiticica, set up situations in the early sixties which were aimed directly at the sensual perception of natural objects or of other people. It was characteristic of such art that it could only be experienced through taking part: the artist offered a situation and the rest was up to a public who could not remain passive. There were hints here of the contemporary move towards group therapy: people finding some kind of release from an urban environment by letting the sand of Oiticica's environments run through their fingers and toes, or breaking through the mental barriers that prevent physical contact between strangers by manipulating Lydia Clark's simple encounter devices for head and hands. Such events, like those arranged by David Medalla and John Dugger, shared the naïve and innocent character of participation art, much of which passed directly into community-orientated activities.

The experience of modern psychiatry, psychology and group therapy have found their way into the cooler and more objective performance art of a number of young American artists, among them Vito Acconci, Dennis Oppenheim and Terry Fox. The exposure of areas of taboo in modern society has formed a central part of the long-

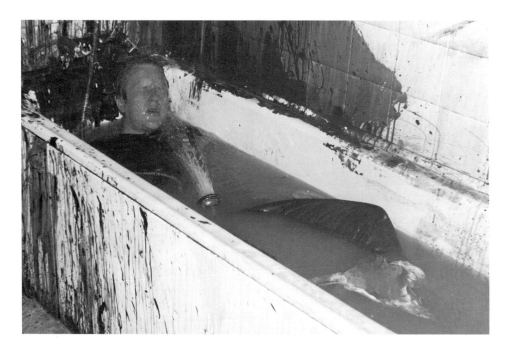

Stuart Brisley in a bath of offal: *And for Today –
Nothing*. Action at Gallery House, London, 1972.

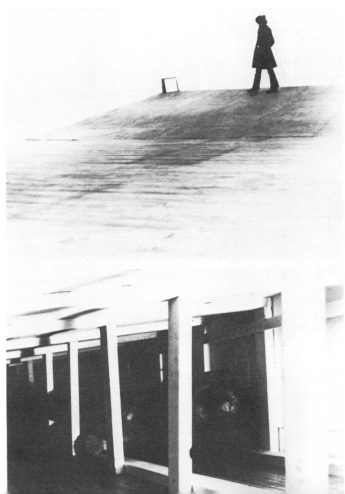

Vito Acconci, *Seedbed*. The spectator, or rather
voyeur, could only hear the artist, who was
underneath the wooden ramp, noisily
masturbating.

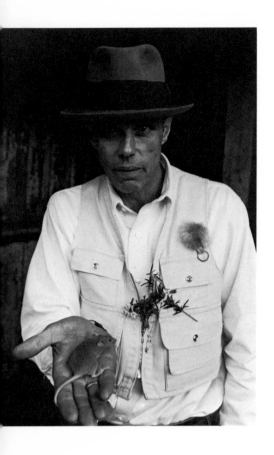

Joseph Beuys with a mouse, linking 'the higher senses and the lower senses', during the filming of *How Does it Feel?*

suffering art of Vito Acconci, who takes the areas of behaviour that are usually kept private or suppressed, say sexual and masturbatory activity or the manifestations of paranoia, and re-enacts them in public. *Seedbed* was such a performance. The audience knew that the artist as masturbator was there under the wooden ramp over which they walked in the gallery. They were aware of his presence under their feet through the sounds of his activity. Acconci's intention was to create the tension needed to make what he terms 'the powerfield' perceptible. At the same time the audience was inevitably reminded of the essentially voyeuristic nature of the passive art public, and of the distance that separates the doer from the beholder, whatever the medium. Dennis Oppenheim uses his own body as a measure of physical and psychological phenomena. Works recorded photographically, like those of so many of these artists, range from the simple demonstration of the pigment changes caused by exposing areas of the body to sun and heat to more complex human situations, often involving transfer of experience: Oppenheim traced a drawing with his finger on his son's back; simultaneously the child attempted to transfer this felt but unseen drawing on to the wall in front of him.

While artists like Acconci and Oppenheim use their own bodies as instruments of measurement for the spatial projection of psychological phenomena, Terry Fox, like Joseph Beuys with whom he has worked, attempts to regain a position of synthesis between body and spirit sometimes through practices reminiscent of shamanism. Fox's art, with its emphasis on reaching areas of experience beyond the restrictions of the body, is a direct attempt to change the consciousness of the spectator, and his performances are not easily reduced to words. They have, for instance, focused the attention on the simple beauty of a fish and the vibrations of its life as they were transmitted via strings to Fox's own body. He has demonstrated the energies that are present in the most familiar objects: the heat energy of an electric light bulb speeding up the burning of a lighted candle, or the mysterious passage of smoke over the body.

The perception and generation of energy is a key to some of the most stimulating activities of recent years. It implies an art that appeals to the senses as a whole rather than separately. It also changes the emphasis from the completion of single works presented as finished entities to the idea of life/art as an ongoing activity. The time sense becomes increasingly important both for continuity and in the process of accumulating experience. Some artists, like the Italian Pierpaolo Calzolari, find they can plough layer upon layer of perception of energy and tension back into a performance that can be constantly repeated in modified or extended forms. Paul Neagu, a Rumanian working in London, presents his work as a process of growth and of transition from one kind of energy to the next in a steadily rising spiral of intensity. Both Calzolari and Neagu have used blindfolds in order to increase inner psychological awareness of other peoples' presence and movements. For Calzolari, the body is a monitor or gauge of psychological tension; for Neagu it is a transmitter of energy.

Two things should be said at this point. First, there's a paradox in this general movement towards a more direct and sensual art. It's not purely based on instinct and feeling. Many of the artists discussed have more than a layman's knowledge of the fields brought together in this book. The work of the last ten years can be seen as the beginning of a wider form of research, and its formulation is still in many cases at its primitive stages. The second point is related: the wider definition of art proposed by such activities was born of a dissatisfaction with the limited potential of the static art object and its museum or gallery context that was fairly widespread in the sixties. The search for alternatives may have taken the artist into psychological, sociological, anthropological or linguistic fields, but he still has to have a means and a form for processing his findings back into art. Many have turned to performance, film, photography or video to do so. Some have sought alternatives in the field of community art, leaving the gallery circuit for a licensed form of social therapy directed towards encouraging the participation of a society that lives through second-hand sensory experience. But the object remains important. Man, after all, will always process his encounter with material into some form, and will continue to feel the need to do so. Brancusi's *Birth of the World: Sculpture for the Blind*, a simple egg shape that contradicts Plato's dismissal of the sense of touch by appealing directly to the spirit through the senses, remains an important example, and a balance to the influence of Duchamp, his friend and contemporary. *The Birth of the World* is a demonstration of timelessness beyond changing style in art: a simple form shaped by man that evokes the source and mystery of life.

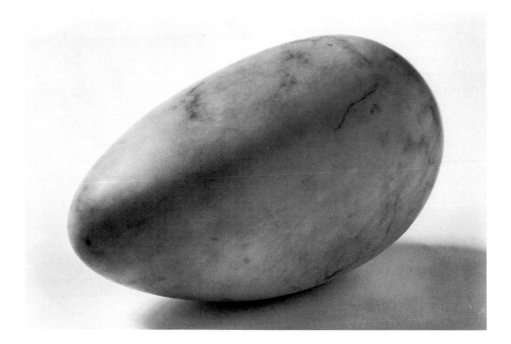

Constantin Brancusi, *Birth of the World: Sculpture for the Blind*.

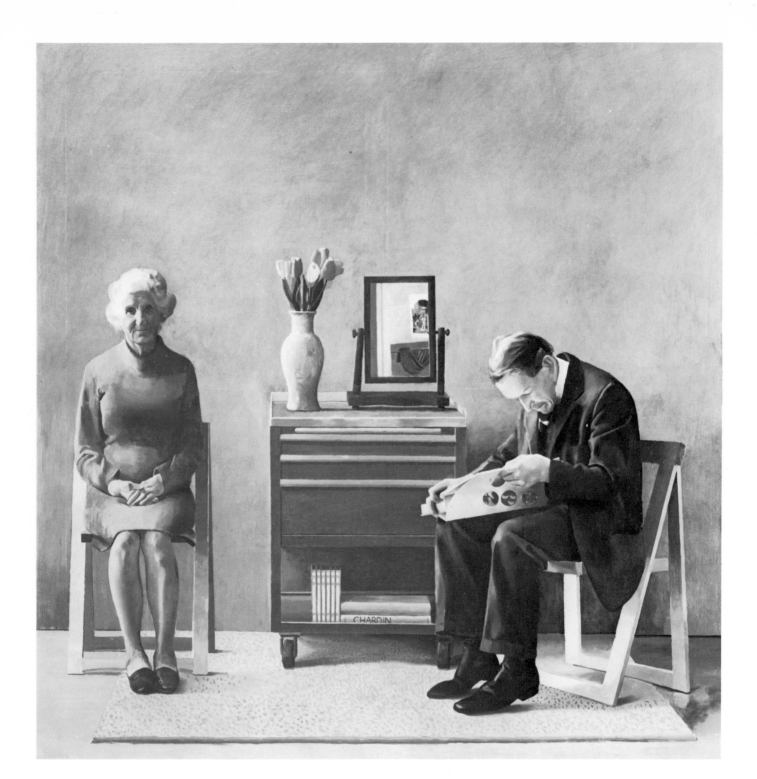

DAVID HOCKNEY

David Hockney is one of the most widely known British painters at work today. In addition to his representational and characteristically witty portraits he has produced many hundreds of drawings and prints. He has also designed three highly acclaimed stage productions: *Ubu Roi* (1966), *The Rake's Progress* (1975) and *The Magic Flute* (1978).

Painting a picture

Four years ago I decided I would paint my parents. I wondered how I was going to do it. It was not easy at all. I kept putting it off. I actually began it about fourteen months ago, when I was in Paris. I wondered if they should be in their little house in Bradford, surrounded by their furniture, the things they have. Then I decided to place them in my own environment, although it has nothing to do with them. All the objects on the trolley are mine: the little mirror, the photograph album, the picture books of paintings and the four volumes of Proust. Tulips are my favourite flowers. I have always ignored the background. I thought it was not necessary to put in the wallpaper; it would be superfluous.

I have done five or six double portraits before. Doing my parents is the most complex challenge to date. It is a psychological study. I have to look at myself a little more when doing it. I realized I should literally do just that in the picture, so I put myself in the mirror on the trolley as though it was reflecting me looking at them. I have changed myself many times. That is my eighth self-portrait.

My parents are not very articulate people. At first my thoughts were, 'My God, they're not communicating!' They would sit in silence for hours, but then I realized there was some communication – something else going on that was not verbal. So in the painting I wanted to somehow get the feeling of separateness and silence and communication. There are links in silence. A lot of people have said my pictures are silent. In this particular painting I have worked on that aspect very consciously.

At the moment, the way it is going, the only successful bit is that mood. The floor is a mess. It doesn't quite work. If I got it to work it would make the mood even stronger. I think it is just beginning to work. There is something there.

I think it is good to follow the senses. It is good to trust your intuition, which of course not many people do; they think it is difficult. I thought it was easy because I have always trusted mine, but I slowly realized that most people don't. That's all part of trusting your senses.

Learning to draw is learning to develop a visual sense. I went to a very old-fashioned academic art school for four years. All I did was draw from a nude model. Doing that makes you look very carefully and interpret in line or tone or colour. I think it is a very good education for anybody. It is being forced to look at something carefully that is good, not the finished drawing.

David Hockney, *My Parents*, 1976.

149

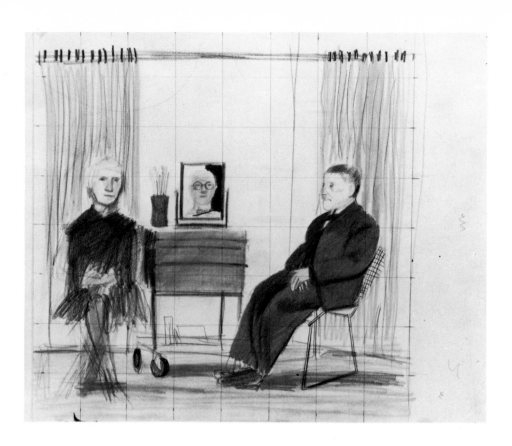

Pencil sketch for the 1975 version, opposite.

I do a lot of drawing with colour and tone, but I think line-drawing is the most superior. It is much more difficult to reduce form and volume and feeling to a line. The intellectual work is much greater. It is not easy to do. When I am making a line-drawing I am very tense all the time. If music is on I don't hear it. I am sitting on the edge of my chair all the time, with my back off. I can't move either way to rest until I have finished the drawing. It is very exciting, but it is also incredibly tiring. I can't do it all day. The tension is a bit too much.

The imaginative use of the senses is the interesting thing. Everybody has senses, but they don't put them to imaginative use. Incidentally, I have tried a number of drugs because I think any imaginative person should, but now I tend to think that I am permanently higher than lots of people who take drugs. I can feel excited all of the time without drugs, but I can understand people wanting a kind of adventure. What I cannot understand is why official opposition to drugs cannot take all this into account. I think everybody is entitled to his own adventure in life. My adventure is art and if anybody tried to rob me of it I would fight like mad. Unfortunately people in authority lack imagination in that they can't see that they are having their adventure. For instance even today a politician will refer to his 'sense of duty' – well,

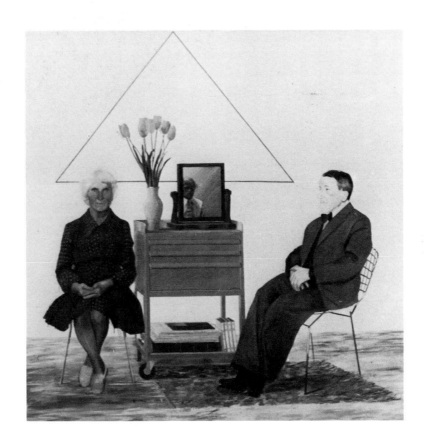

David Hockney, *My Parents and Myself*, 1975.

Detail from the 1975 version: self-portrait in the mirror.

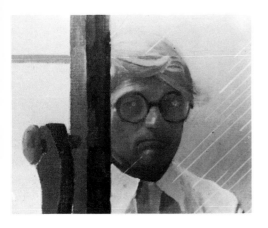

that's balls; they are having a good time, an adventure. They are entitled to their adventure, but if only they had a little more imagination they could understand that other people also want an adventure and it might be in a very different area.

I choose to make pictures because I love pictures. They make my experience of life more vivid. They are a wonderful way of communicating my own feelings and observations to other people. Of course they only work if I succeed in getting something across to somebody else. If nobody gets anything I have failed, however beautifully I have painted the subject.

I have always thought that my paintings have content; they are never just about the painting itself. I have always thought that great pictures, great art, is always about the human figure. In fact the lines from W. H. Auden's poem 'Letter to Lord Byron' say it very sympathetically:

> To me art's subject is the human clay
> And landscape but a background to a torso
> All Cézanne's apples I would give away
> For a Goya or a Daumier.

151

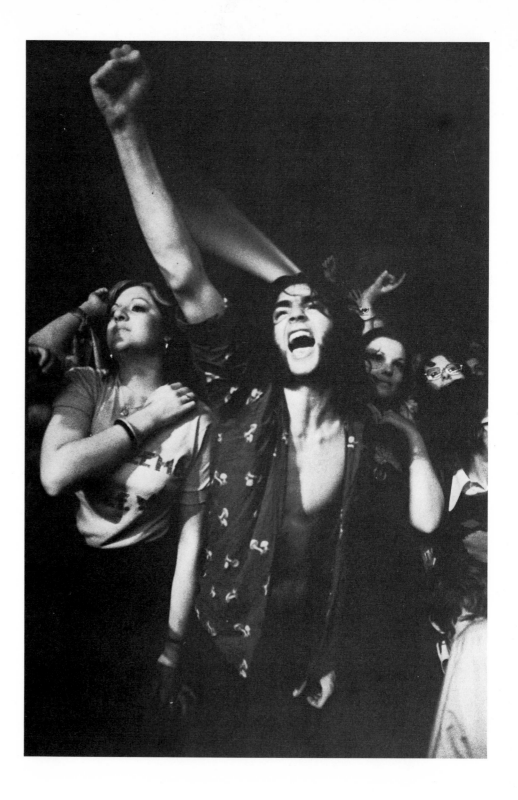

MICK GOLD

Mick Gold has written, and illustrated with his own photographs, *Rock on the Road*. His theme is rock music's ability, as a major industry, to put people into touch with their senses and feelings by making them listen, look, dance, think and feel.

See me, feel me, touch me, heal me.
from Rock Opera *Tommy*

STOP

Help Save The Youth of America
DON'T BUY NEGRO RECORDS

(If you don't want to serve negroes in your place of business, then do not have negro records on your juke box or listen to negro records on the radio.)

The screaming, idiotic words, and savage music of these records are undermining the morals of our white youth in America.

Call the advertisers of the radio stations that play this type of music and complain to them!

Don't Let Your Children Buy, or Listen
To These Negro Records

Rock music and the senses

Contemporary Western culture excels at dividing our minds from our bodies, sexual activity from cerebral, serious 'art' from popular 'entertainment', the act of creation from the industry of consumption. Separate areas are allotted to analytic thought, to emotional indulgence, to physical energy. The truly difficult task is to integrate these activities. I believe this has been rock music's real importance in our society: by creating a popular art that could make you think *and* dance *and* feel, rock has healed some of the divisions between our minds and our bodies, between private experiences and public values. But the elements that were eventually synthesized within rock music stretch back into the archaeology of Western culture, along with the taboos and repressions that the music tried to confront.

The slave trade transported the polyrhythms of Africa to the New World. Tens of thousands of blacks were carried like cattle across the Atlantic. In the cotton fields of Mississippi, they developed a call-and-response style of work song: the leader called out the lines, the labourers replied with the chorus. This collective form of folk music co-ordinated the work of cotton pickers and prison gangs, and, to some extent, helped to lighten their back-breaking toil beneath the noonday sun.

Although these African rhythms were mixed with other musical forms that the blacks encountered – jigs and reels from Scotland and Ireland, *contredanses* from France – the music still embodied a profound cultural schism: white society possessed the brains, blacks possessed the brawn. The American Negro had been condemned by history to providing the muscle-power for the cotton plantations and, later, for the wartime expansion of the industrial sector. As a result of this schism, however, blacks were also endowed with an aura of super-sexuality, an aura that inspired both contempt and fascination in the white society of the deep South. In the vitality of the music which accompanied their work patterns, their evening recreation, their religious services, was a spirit of resilience, a simple sensual pleasure which frequently masked their embittered and ironic feelings towards American society. Black music frequently aroused fear in white society; it was a fear of the body, fear of the unspoken bargains that bound society together, arising out of an almost unconscious creed of white puritanism. Echoes of this fear were frequently heard during the early years of rock 'n' roll.

153

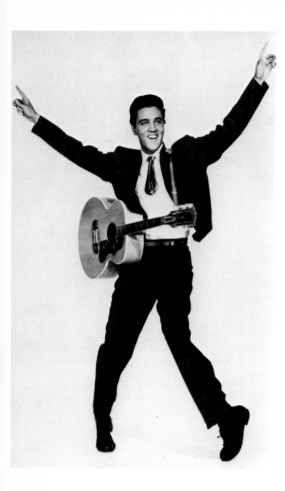

Elvis Presley.

Songs of Innocence

So Elvis Presley came, strumming a weird guitar and wagging his tail across the continent, ripping off fame and fortune as he scrunched his way and, like a latterday Johnny Appleseed, sowing seeds of a new rhythm and style in the white souls of the white youth of America, whose inner hunger and need was no longer satisfied.

Soul on Ice, Eldridge Cleaver

Musically, Elvis Presley married white country and western music, melodic and sentimental, with black rhythm and blues, abrasive and sensual. In August 1954 his first recording coupled 'That's Alright Mama', an uptempo R & B number, with 'Blue Moon of Kentucky', a blue-grass hit. The initial response to Presley's sound was confusion, but the long-term effects were earth-shaking. What Presley's first record symbolized was a bridge across one of the great divides of popular culture, linking 'love' with sex. Songs for white audiences, peddled by crooners with big bands backing them, tended to idealize and romanticize, transforming sexual energy into a symbolic code. 'Fly me to the moon and let me play among the stars,' warbled Frank Sinatra politely. On the other side of the musical tracks, in the black R & B charts, Hank Ballard sang 'Work With Me Annie' and Muddy Waters drawled 'I Just Want To Make Love To You', honest music powered by an infectious back-beat and amplified guitars.

The stage performances of Frank Sinatra and Johnny Ray, the former characterized by avalanches of fainting fans, the latter by exercises in emotional overkill, had revealed audiences anxious for stronger material than that provided by the crooner/big band brand of popular music. Finally, Elvis Presley took the lid off the musical orgone box. He was helped by the post-war proliferation and sophistication of the media, which enabled him to storm America on a national scale. His concerts caused riots, radio stations broadcast his insidious new sound across the land, but perhaps television was his most important ally. Adults immediately sensed how subversive he was from the *way* he sang: 'For the ear he is an unutterable bore, not nearly as talented as Frank Sinatra . . . nor does he convey the emotional fury of a Johnny Ray. From watching Mr Presley it is wholly evident that his skill lies in another direction. His one speciality is an accented movement of the body that heretofore has been primarily identified with the blonde bombshell of the burlesque runway. The gyration never had anything to do with the world of popular music and still doesn't.' This was the verdict of Jack Gould, television critic of the *New York Times*, in June 1956. Significantly, the next time that Presley appeared on American TV, the cameras only filmed him from the waist up.

James Dean had been the teenage icon of internalized anguish: misinterpreted, mistrusted, mumbling and vulnerable. It was rock 'n' roll, via Presley, which externalized that energy. The mid-fifties party was brief but noisy: 'Tin Pan Alley has unleashed a new monster, a nightmare of rhythm. Some of our disc jockeys have put emotional TNT on their turntables. Rock 'n' roll gives young hoodlums an excuse to get together. It inflames teenagers and is obscenely suggestive,' announced one district attorney in Massachusetts, over newspaper accounts of demolished concert halls and teenage stabbings.

If Presley was the body, it was Chuck Berry who added brains to the first wave of rock energy. He could do the duckwalk (a spectacularly stylized movement whereby the singer appeared to float across the stage with one leg constantly horizontal) while enunciating the slyest, bitter-sweet satires on teenage life-styles ever written. In Berry's songs, car bodies and women's bodies were interchangeable, while his guitar riffs described the epic American sense of freedom and constant motion. He created anthems out of lovingly detailed accounts of cult cars, highway towns, soft drinks and high-school mores; his musical energy made the audience move, while his lyrics acknowledged the plasticity and ephemerality of teen culture without compromising the music's *joie de vivre*:

> Sweet little sixteen, she's got the grown-up blues;
> Tight dresses and lipstick, she's sportin' high-heeled shoes;
> Oh but tomorrow morning, she'll have to change her trend
> And be sweet sixteen back in class again.

The fact that Chuck Berry's songs could be both naïve and knowing, both dance rhythms and self-satire, suggested that the split between the mind and body of rock culture was not as absolute as rock 'n' roll's hysterical opponents had assumed.

Tales of Power

> I'm ready to go anywhere, I'm ready for to fade
> Into my own parade, cast your dancing spell my way
> I promise to go under it.
>
> 'Mr Tambourine Man', Bob Dylan

In the fifties, rock 'n' roll had offered vitality in a sterile social landscape. The music articulated the pressures of city life, and from its rhythms created anthems that gave young people a sense of their own power. In the sixties, the music aspired to fuse this physical energy with political protest and imaginative explorations of other realities – to create an alternative consciousness. The most important work in this process was done by the Beatles – 'popular' artists who discovered that they had minds of their own – and by Bob Dylan, a 'serious' artist who discovered that he had a body.

Dylan's first recordings were rooted in the American folk-blues tradition, and used this form to express the idealism of his campus audiences: denunciations of racism and economic exploitation. But despite the searing intensity of Dylan's imagination and imagery, his music remained a legacy from pre-war, rural American culture, in danger of becoming an anachronism. In Britain, young musicians, such as the Animals and the Rolling Stones, were borrowing from the post-war music of black

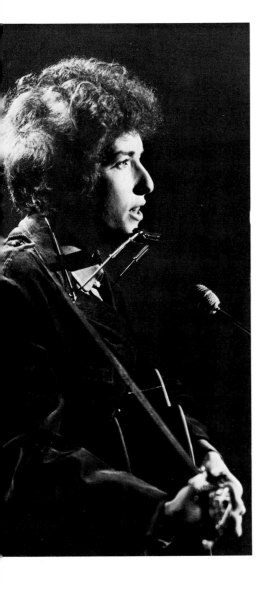

Bob Dylan.

155

America and adapting it to express their own alienation and pent-up energy. Dylan was impressed by the results and set out to create a style which combined the poetry and eloquence of folk-blues with the visceral impact of electric music.

'Like a Rolling Stone' was the hit single that transformed Dylan, in the public imagination, from a finger-pointing folk singer into a surreal rock 'n' roll star. Instead of asking general questions about political problems, his lyrics were more direct: 'How does it *feel?*' he bellowed again and again against a background of cascading organ chords and jagged guitars which thundered like a demonic waterfall, inundating the listener. A deluge of sensory impressions was implicit in Dylan's account of how he wrote the song:

> It was ten pages long. It wasn't called anything, just a rhythm thing on paper – all about my steady hatred directed at some point that was honest. . . . It was telling someone they didn't know what it was all about and they were lucky. I had never thought of it as a song until one day I was at the piano, and on the paper it was singing 'How does it feel?' in the utmost of slow motion. It was like swimming in lava. Hanging by their arms from a birch tree. Skipping, kicking the tree, hitting a nail with your foot. Seeing someone in the pain they were bound to meet up with. I wrote it. I didn't fail. It was straight.

The Beatles also began with the body rhythms of black music, but their sound was more melodic and less threatening than the Rolling Stones'. Also the way in which the Beatles operated as a group, psychologically as well as musically, presented the

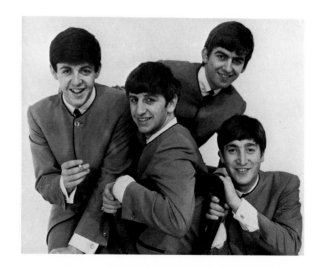

The Beatles.

public with an extraordinary mythic image of integration. McCartney was versatile and charming, Lennon was sarcastic and unpredictable, Harrison was aloof and introverted, and Ringo was unpretentious and stolid. Round and round they went, one body with four heads which never settled into a rut and never ran out of energy.

The Beatles' music began as an ingenious amalgamation of the call-and-response style of gospel groups with the harsher rhythms of rock 'n' roll; what brought their songs to life was their subtle grasp of vernacular speech and an instinct for breaking out of formulae – injecting slang, slurring words across several beats, creating unorthodox bridge passages. Lennon and McCartney's flair for speech rhythms enabled them to create richly emotive effects out of basic English. But then the Beatles wearied of the hysterical adulation that accompanied their public performances and withdrew from the spotlight. They decided that they were serious artists, experimented with drugs, laboured in the recording studio for 700 hours and reincarnated themselves as 'Sgt Pepper's Lonely Hearts Club Band': their sound had become more ethereal, moving from the body to the brain, utilizing orchestras, echo, phasing, sound effects – techniques which made 'Sgt Pepper' resemble the sound track for a vision, rather than simple beat music. And the characters who inhabited this vision included circus acrobats, old-age pensioners, mystics, traffic wardens, misunderstood parents: the 'Sgt Pepper' record was an integrated work which gestured towards a far wider view of society than the narcissism of teenage culture. No one could dance to it; it was a formal statement to be interpreted and analysed. It was the key event which made rock music believe it had evolved into a platform for an alternative consciousness.

The Lonely Hearts Club was a good metaphor for what young people looked for in their music: an asylum for those who felt alienated from the family or society they happened to be born into. Inside the Club, the major preoccupations were magic, drugs, time and space travel, mysticism, oneness with nature – any alternative to materialist, analytic modes of measuring the universe.

Inside the dance halls of San Francisco, at the Avalon and the Fillmore, in the U.F.O. club in London, sound and light crews were transforming music into a total sensory environment. With the aid of sophisticated sound systems, oil slides, film clips, light shows, fire and dry ice, music and visions were integrated and amplified. Internal landscapes were projected outwards. In part, these experiments were a populist acting out of McLuhan's ideas – a belief that all media were extensions of our sensory faculties. They also testified to the fact that music was the one unifying force within the 'underground', a very mixed cocktail containing Buddhism and black magic, political theories and fairy tales, soft and hard drugs.

The music is your special friend
Dance on fire as it intends
Music is your only friend ... until The End.

'The End', The Doors

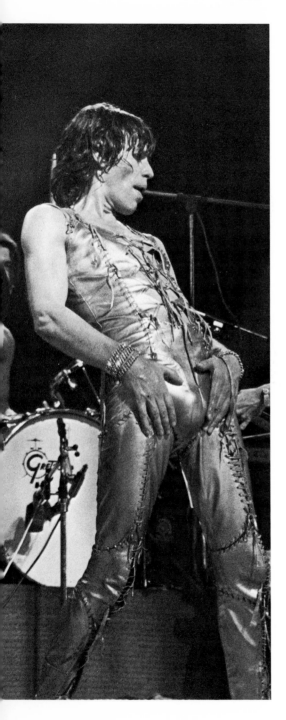
Mick Jagger.

Rock music expanded beyond the confines of the three-minute song. Electronic manipulation created sounds that were akin to the perceptual distortions induced by drugs. A variety of other musical forms – from ragas through reggae to ragtime – were annexed and added to the musical vocabulary of rock; the potential of lengthy improvisation was introduced from jazz, providing musicians with freer expressive possibilities. Rock music became a global village of aural sensations, a sufficiently elastic form to adapt to the shifts of the magpie philosophy which it articulated. No longer restricted to the 'entertainment' category of parties and weekends, the music sought to underpin an entire life-style. All that was now needed was a setting where people could act out the implications of the music in idyllic surroundings, a Garden of Eden wired for sound. In other words, a rock festival.

All the dizzying social and symbolic aspirations of rock music reached their climax in a field in Bethel, New York, in August 1969 when half a million people attended the first 'Aquarian exposition of the arts', the Woodstock Festival. The legend arose that here the musicians, their audience and the rural setting actually did come together and generate a more humane, a more imaginative, a more joyful society. Out of logistical chaos, the event had been transformed into a free festival; everyone worked together to overcome problems of food, transport and health, all drawing strength from the utopian energy embodied in the music.

We are stardust, we are golden
We are billion year old carbon
And we've got to get ourselves back to the Garden
'Woodstock', Joni Mitchell

Millions of young people around the world followed this impulse but, instead, found themselves sitting in muddy, overcrowded fields, listening to distorted music being made by almost invisible musicians half a mile away. Often they were charged exorbitant prices for bad food, sanitary conditions quickly became disgusting, and the local police force welcomed the event as an opportunity to boost their tally of drug arrests. The disparity between the myth of Woodstock Nation and the frequently sordid, chaotic reality of rock festivals typified the way in which rock culture ended the sixties by overdosing on its own ideology. Rock music had described the re-unification of physical needs, social values and imaginative possibilities. But the music's victory was an artistic, a symbolic achievement, not easily reconciled with the problems of everyday life. A diet of drugs, magic and music proved to be inadequate protection against the pressures of a competitive, materialist society; it would take much more than a long weekend in the country (which ultimately proved very profitable for record and film companies) to lead the children of the Western industrial world back into that mythical Garden.

Songs of Experience

Oooooooh, isn't it nice
When you find your heart is made out of ice?

'Ride Sally Ride', Lou Reed

In 1967 a New York group, the Velvet Underground, recorded a song about drug addiction. Entitled 'Heroin', it was a totally deadpan account of the situation viewed from the addict's point of view; hints of alienation, self-destruction, a desperation for sensation, surfaced and sank in a black swamp of sound that evoked blood clots building up, tourniquets being tightened, anxieties being dissolved, in a dark and clumsy rush of music:

I don't know where I'm going
But I'm going to try for the kingdom if I can
'Cause it makes me feel like I'm a man
When I put a spike into my veins and
I tell you things aren't quite the same...

'Heroin', Lou Reed

The song bypassed the romanticized accounts of drug experiences being recorded by other underground groups and zeroed in on the street addict, the lowest figure in the drug hierarchy, depicting his situation as starkly as a piece of subway graffiti. During their lifetime (1966–70) the Velvet Underground sold few records, and remained unknown to the mass public. But during the seventies, Lou Reed (who wrote all their songs) has exerted a powerful influence on younger rock musicians. As rock's utopian aspirations became more and more unbelievable, Reed's realistic canvases of city life provided a more credible alternative. But his influence was subtler than that. It was his style, his sensibility, that invited emulation. His cool observations and ability to extract vitality from a fabric of decay and corruption looked like a survival kit for the seventies.

The lesson was not lost on David Bowie, who shared Reed's interest in a demimonde of bisexuality, stylization, and irony. 'Ziggy Stardust', Bowie's rock star persona and his most flamboyant creation, was a lively mixture of science fiction fantasies, androgynous gestures, and jaded idealism. And yet the vision was circumscribed by the self-conscious artificiality of the star's identity – a butterfly creature with a brief life-span. Bowie's adroit manipulation of his own image effectively subverted the political implications of his music.

In the fifties, rock's celebration of physical grace, in dancing and in sexuality, had offered a code which bound 'us', the teenagers, together against 'them', the adults. In the sixties this implicit message was politicized into an explicit set of values, an invocation of alternative realities to which 'we' could flee. By the seventies, the music had become both too established and too fragmentary to maintain such a pose: a variety of us's, against each other. Undeniably a branch of show business,

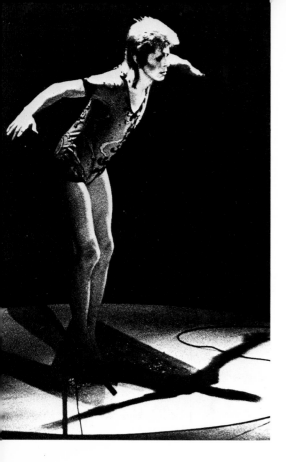

David Bowie.

rather than a guerrilla counter-culture. And there were no totemic figures, such as Presley or Dylan, to give unity to its message. While some musicians offered nostalgic pastiches of rock's past achievements as an escape from contemporary fragmentation, others re-examined the past more critically.

The Pink Floyd's music successfully synthesized such classic, romantic themes as nostalgia for childhood, empathy with nature, a sense of loss, with the science-fiction implications of their complex stage technology. The lyrics of their albums became preoccupied with the ways in which society penalizes deviancy, describing how spiritual and imaginative pursuits are eroded by the need for financial and emotional security, how the record business can transform visionary energy into industrial product. But these rather grim themes were presented with enormous technical panache in the Floyd's concerts. To accompany 'The Dark Side Of The Moon''s aura of incipient madness, batteries of speakers whirled the sound around the auditorium; footsteps, echoes, and screams besieged the audience from all sides; surreal cinematic montages flowed from a giant screen above the group; waves of dry ice shrouded the Floyd beneath banks of fog. Yet their shows had developed from the random sensory barrage of the early psychedelic clubs into a subtler, more structured event. Beneath the superficial dazzle and disorientation of the Floyd's performances, a classical sense of order and stoic musical dignity had evolved. The richness of their music and the spectacle of their performances summed up the way in which rhythm and blues, electronic experiments, and classical forms, could combine to create sounds that were simultaneously rhythmic yet ethereal, romantic yet contemporary, abstract yet ritualistic, experimental yet profitable.

Inevitably, the sheer extravagance of the Pink Floyd's performances implied a massive distance between the musicians and their audience. The complexity and cost of their equipment emphasized that the major rock musicians lived far away from their subjects – only able to reach them through sound systems transported by chartered jets, surrounded by laser beams, and protected by security forces in their hundreds. Inevitably, the supergroups of the seventies generated a musical antithesis. Its name was Punk Rock.

> I am an anti-Christ
> I am an anarchist
> Don't know what I want but I know how to get it
> I want to destroy passers-by
> 'Cos I wanna be . . . anarchy
>
> 'Anarchy in the U.K.', Jones/Matlock/Cook/Rotten

The clothing that accompanied this music reeked of bondage, mutilation, and fetishism – safety pins, razor blades, ripped shirts and straitjackets. The movement borrowed its styles from the lunatic asylum, the Nazi Party, and the market in fetishized sex; these were combined into an aggressive expression of the ripped-up

160

feelings of an alienated working-class generation. Musically, Punk Rock was fast, loud, and terse; lyrically, it was preoccupied with unemployment, psychotic behaviour, and a sense of social disintegration. In live performances the chief innovations were 'pogo dancing' – leaping up and down in an unstable manner, and 'gobbing' – drowning the performers in a torrent of saliva.

It was difficult to defend this 'New Wave' of music without seeming to endorse nihilism and gratuitous violence. That was half of its meaning. Yet the music also possessed a ferocious honesty, total contempt for the moribund and class-ridden structures of an economically depressed society. Out of its own negativity, the music generated a sense of release. At its very best – as when the Sex Pistols' sarcastic anthem 'God Save the Queen' topped the charts during Queen Elizabeth's Silver Jubilee, while being systematically censored by every major retail chain and radio station – rock music once again legitimized revolt.

Today, rock music has overtaken the film industry in dollar turnover. Elvis's hedonism, Dylan's visions, the Beatles' versatility, always underpinned by the rhythms of black music, have created the wealthiest entertainment empire this world has known. And also the most ubiquitous. In pubs, at parties, in supermarkets, on car radios, in bars and at home, rock music has somehow synthesized everyday speech and the rhythms of the city into an electric art that is the authentic sound of our time. Just when the mass media and industrialization were deemed to be destroying popular culture, replacing it with centralized pre-digested pap, rock has shown itself to be responsive to sub-cultures, to local traditions, and to have some built-in equilibrium: coming back to earth if it becomes too experimental, seeking new sources if it becomes too simplified. And rock has also shown itself to be capable of absorbing some frightening contradictions: maintaining a populist façade while being marketed with all the manipulative slickness of any lucrative consumer product. Rock music remains a form of social energy, rather than poetry or 'pure' music. It does not sit quietly in the corner, observing, passing carefully balanced judgements. Rock music operates at the very heart of the beast of industrial, capitalist society. When it succeeds, it is on a huge, possibly grotesque scale. And that is also the source of its power.

If its recent artistic successes have either been accounts of dead dreams or celebrations of nihilism, that says more about rock's ability to mirror the present, than about its intrinsic message. It is still the sound of vitality, the fetal heartbeat that underlies the music, and that has been its greatest asset in keeping on in a world constantly trying to lose touch with itself.

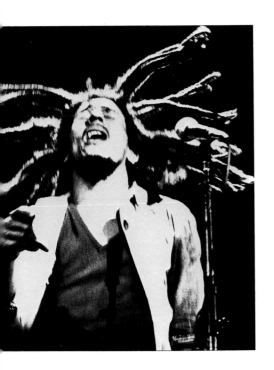

Bob Marley.

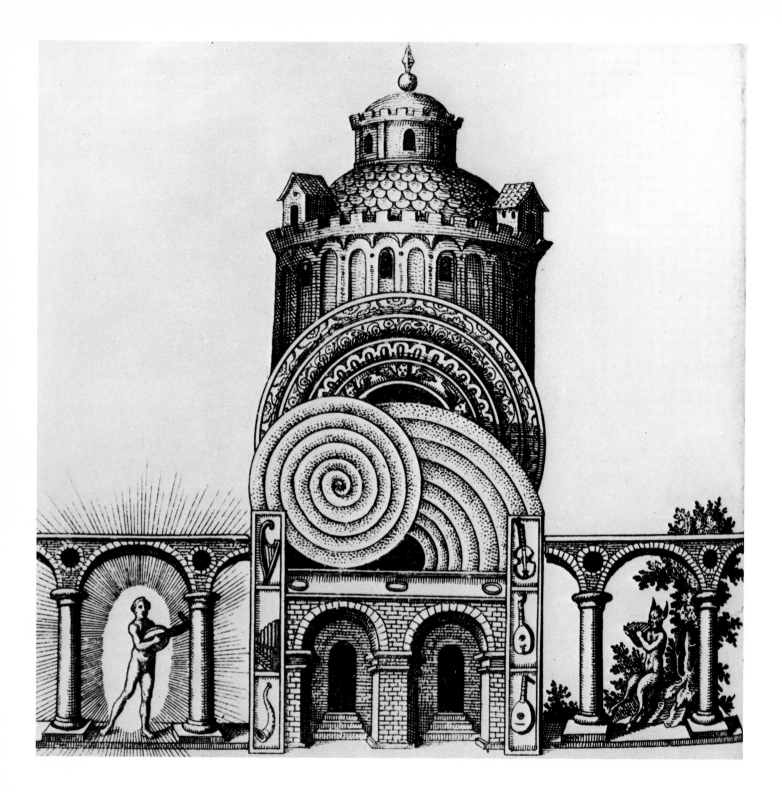

MEIRION BOWEN

Meirion Bowen writes about music and is director of a percussion-music/theatre group. He has made a special study of contemporary American music, especially the work of Harry Partch, and is currently combining music and dance at the London School of Contemporary Dance.

Music of the mind and body

Sound is an auditory phenomenon. Music is something else. Its assimilation and appreciation can and do involve all the senses. A person almost deaf from early childhood (as opposed to, say, a Beethoven, whose deafness came gradually upon him from about his early thirties, when he was already a mature creative musician) is still able to learn to perform music and obtain gratification from the experience of it. Such a person's sense of touch might compensate for inadequate hearing apparatus. The 'feeling' is there, though it has been stimulated or acquired differently. It seems, as such, to be a crystallization of several inter-related processes happening over a period of time – and not only for the duration of the performance: the musicians stop playing, but the music goes on inside us.

In the present epoch, a collision has occurred between the musical attitudes of the West – which have tended towards abstraction – and those characteristics of ethnic cultures, where the physical wellsprings and motivations are overt. It has been a fruitful collision. Each side has learnt from the other. In contemporary music there are thus not only extremes of abstract and gestural music-making, but also an important middle ground where an incredible variety of creative permutations has arisen. My intention in this chapter is to show something of these extremes and delineate some of the different rapprochements that have been attempted.

In all non-Western cultures, music has retained a close connection with physical movement and gesture. Musical expression is thus related to everyday work or play – the songs sung out in a bush village by an African woman pounding maize, or by children in Liverpool's slums as they play in the streets – or it may reflect the desires of individuals and groups for some kind of spiritual or ecstatic state of being – Negro church services that develop from the call-and-response of preacher and congregation into virtual jam sessions. All this survives up to the present day. It contrasts with the Western tradition, wherein an alternative mode has been cultivated, involving musical expression as an object or artefact separate from the physical means of its production. This move in the direction of abstraction has both fascinated and repelled Western musical exponents and audiences.

This doesn't mean that all music-making in the West has been characterized by cold detachment for a few hundred years – far from it! We need cite only two fairly colourful instances where the opposite is in fact patently obvious.

Music of the mind and body symbolically represented by Robert Fludd in *Metaphysica*, 1617.

163

Anton Schindler, Beethoven's biographer, tells of a visit he made to the composer during the composition (in 1819) of the *Missa Solennis*:

> In the living-room, which was locked, we heard the master singing parts of the fugue in the 'Credo' – singing, howling, stamping. After listening to this almost terrifying performance for a long time, we were about to leave when the door opened, and Beethoven stood before us, his features so distorted that it was enough to inspire fear. . . . His first utterances were confused, as if he had been disagreeably surprised by our overhearing him.

Wagner's need for a background of silks, satins, furs and perfumes in which to live and work was partly the result of a skin allergy, yet he found it hard to compose in any other environment. This strange compulsion reached fetishistic heights during the creation of *Parsifal* in the late 1870s. Wagner's latest *amour*, Judith Gautier, had to send him boundless quantities of amber, Milk of Iris (he poured half a bottle of it into his daily bath) and Rose de Bengale; and he asked for powdered scents to sprinkle over fabrics. His study in Wahnfried was immediately above the bathroom, and as he sat working in his silk and fur outfits, he breathed in the exotic aromas that wafted up from below.

The *Missa Solennis* and *Parsifal* can be understood independently of their respective creators' lives, yet their production involved the entire physical being and senses of the latter. (Wagner's music-drama ideal entailed the domination of the audience's whole sensory responses by the works performed; but that is a separate issue.)

Opinion is somewhat divided as to exactly how much histrionics can be tolerated from players, singers and conductors, and to what extent such behaviour is essential to the full enjoyment of a performance. The same temperament will often find acceptable Beecham's flamboyance and Boult's self-effacement, Kreisler's wayward caprice and Heifetz's steely strength. For the assumption is that ultimately the musical results can be judged *apart* from the manner of their production; the very existence of the hi-fi industry seems to reinforce this assumption, whether it be true or not.

During the last 200 years or so, it was above all *instrumental* music which, in the West, was more and more considered to possess those mysterious powers of suggestion for which music could be valued very highly. Profound and thorough exploration of its formal and linguistic potential might even provide the key to some hidden order in the universe. Hence some have come to believe that its sister science must be mathematics, and the arrival of the computer has brought the activities of musical composition and mathematical investigation actually under the same roof.

We have here virtually a revival of the Renaissance notion (derived from the Greeks) that music existed not only in everyday practical manifestations, but as a

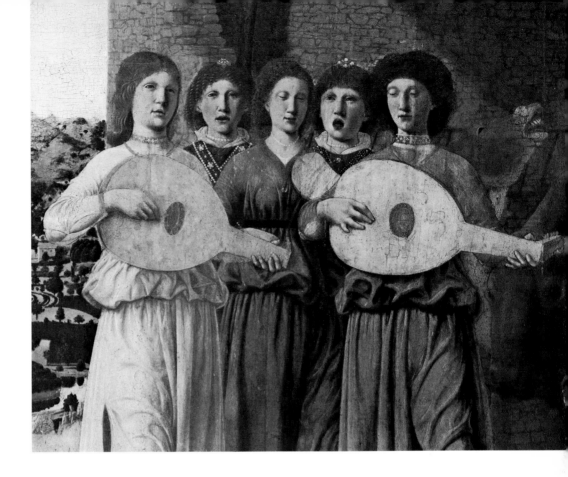

branch of philosophical speculation, as a metaphor, in fact, for some divine plan in the universe – hence the idea of 'the music of the spheres'. But then, unlike now, the most elevated form of music-making was thought to be vocal, since the process of tying music closely to words ensured the didactic and moral value of the end result, whereas purely instrumental music was suspect: it could arouse and excite the passions to an uncontrollable degree, and maybe to immoral ends. In this context, vocal polyphony and accompanied songs (e.g. lute-songs) were esteemed most highly.

With the development of the modern orchestra and of instruments capable of great flexibility and variety of expression, the position of purely instrumental music changed. It became an alternative medium for dramatic composition for those composers (e.g. Beethoven and Berlioz) whose operatic ambitions were constantly being thwarted. It was still an object of suspicion. Beethoven and Berlioz managed to draw an audience (and a new *concert*-going audience at that) for their symphonies. But Beethoven's string quartets were for decades thought eccentric, unplayable and unacceptable as chamber music compositions by most music-lovers, other than small groups of cognoscenti. In the operahouse, to give the orchestra too extensive a

Angels singing carols: detail of Piero della Francesca's *Nativity*.

role was controversial: remember Mozart's *Die Entführung aus dem Serail*, of which the Emperor Joseph said, 'Too beautiful for our ears, and a prodigious lot of notes, dear Mozart'; or Wagner, who was always under attack for the way the orchestra dominated the attention, swamping the voices and all the other elements in his music-dramas. Nevertheless, during the nineteenth century in Europe there developed a new attitude. Berlioz writing a treatise on orchestration, Liszt and Chopin establishing the grand piano as a kind of orchestra in its own right – these were influential forces enabling instrumental music to be considered eventually as the prime vehicle for musical abstraction. Towards the close of the nineteenth century music had become, for many artists, the supreme art, by virtue of its self-sufficiency – the capacity of instrumental music to stand apart, yet also to embrace (or so it seemed) all the other arts. In the Symbolist movement of the 1880s and 1890s, all the arts aspired to the abstract condition of instrumental music. In turn, instrumental music stimulated theories of synaesthesia.

Such supremacy as was accorded to instrumental music is still implicitly accepted in our own epoch by a figure such as Pierre Boulez, and he is a direct heir to the Symbolist movement. It might be illuminating to suggest a parallel between Boulez's creative work and the early *Tractatus* of the philosopher Wittgenstein. With both, the ideal to be attained is the gradual revelation of an abstract substructure to language, purged of all its impurities (which derive from the vernacular, from physically induced modifications and inflexions of speech-sounds and rhythms). The musical end-product with Boulez exhibits an almost fleshless structure. All influences (e.g. Debussy, Messiaen, Stravinsky, Webern, oriental music) have lost their original identity and are submerged beneath a formal outline characterized by a kind of frozen perfection. To ask, 'How does it feel?' in relation to *Le manteau sans maître* (1954) or *Pli selon pli* (1961–8) is to beg many questions. For the apparatus of feeling seems irrelevant. Or nearly so: it is a question of priorities. If a molecular biologist were to attach prime importance to the sheer *beauty* of the processes which he is able to reveal in cellular growth and interaction, he might be criticized, justifiably, for lop-sided values, though no one would deny the validity of his emotional reaction towards what he had discovered. A composer like Boulez is in the position – possibly less socially responsible than that of the scientific worker – of displacing all our primal responses regarding musical experience in favour of the recognition of certain formal characteristics. He wants 'feeling' to become something transcendent, far removed from the commonplace emotions of fear, love and erotic excitement, anxiety and anticipation, nostalgic longings and sadness. It is a superhuman task. Even Boulez had to admit of some reconciliation with, for instance, archetypal expressions of grief and homage when he wrote his *Ritual: in memoriam Maderna* (1975).

Whereas Boulez has been prepared to accept that the public at large can only gradually come to assimilate the implications of complete abstraction in music, and has identified himself with the task of educating them to that end, others in the same (or comparable) field have stood apart. Milton Babbitt, the archpriest of the abstract musical aesthetic in the USA, has pursued compositional goals as if they were entirely and exclusively scientific considerations. He would maintain that his first duty as composer is to his art, to the evolution of music and new musical concepts. He maintains, however, that such concepts are no more for the average man than the advanced theories of astrophysics. His actual music, as it developed from the extension of Webern's technique of pitch organization to other dimensions of music, took him away from the world of human beings as such. For human performers were too fallible and electronics far more dependable. At Princeton University, Babbitt has taught mathematics as well as music, and he sees his own creative work as an ascetic exercise in research, as such producing 'special music in an alien and inapposite world':

> I dare suggest that the composer would do himself and his music an immediate and eventual service by total, resolute and voluntary withdrawal from this public world to one of private performance and electronic media, with its very real possibility of complete elimination of the public and social aspects of musical composition. By so doing, the separation between the domains would be defined beyond any possibility of confusion of categories, and the composer would be free to pursue a private life of professional achievement, as opposed to a public life of unprofessional compromise and exhibitionism.

Abstraction in music is only one aspect which a number of artists in this century have found it necessary to explore to its outer limits. Comparable extremes can be found with music that is generated from and allied with overt bodily expression. Rock 'n' roll swept to success in the late 1950s undoubtedly because, as a genre of popular music, it entailed and invited uninhibited and sometimes hysterical jubilation. Shouting, yelling, screaming, bodily gyrations and 'glossolalia' – an elaborate melisma of vocal sounds, ecstatic and primitive in character – allied to a bombardment of *amplified* instrumental sound: these are the prime features of a musical experience intended directly to accommodate the human being as whole – mind, heart, body. The 'image' of the rock star is as important as what he or she sings or plays – and in a whole category of cases, *more* important then the actual music. Clothes and charisma count for a lot. For in all instances, the audience must be made to feel close to the star, whose dress is similar, or who appears freakishly, surrealistically, as a fantasy-projection of the audience.

Common to the rock world and to the avant-garde now is the evolution of new forms of theatrical presentation within which music no longer remains abstracted or separated from its audience. In the early days of psychedelic pop it entailed an accumulation of musical and visual data without much regard to their precise overall effect. But this has now shaped the entire gamut of presentation in this sphere. The wealthiest stars aim for the most extravagant mixed-media performance wherein no gimmickry is spared to engage the audience wholly in the musical and general artistic 'trip'. Likewise, numerous experiments in what is called 'music-theatre', in Britain, Europe and the USA, have sought to break down the traditional dichotomy between audience and performers. The dividing-line between what is 'pop' and what is 'serious' now becomes impossible to define at all, other than in terms of the type of promotional backing and financial support the performances receive.

A fascinating borderline case is that of the American composer Harry Partch (1901–74), who is better known among the students and hippies in the USA than in academic music circles. Partch received very little subsidy for his endeavours until he was well into his forties. Nevertheless, he stubbornly sought out alternatives to the abstract traditions of European culture. Californian by birth, he was most influenced by the ritual theatre of ancient Greece, by Chinese and Japanese theatrical traditions, and by the rituals of the Mexican Indians. He characterized his music as 'corporeal' as opposed to 'abstract', with its basis in the rhythms and inflections of speech and song, and in movement and dance.

In its early stages, Partch's work concentrated on recitation of poetry to a single-line musical accompaniment (an idea which impressed W. B. Yeats in the 1930s). In the last twenty-five years of his life, Partch developed his ideas in terms of dance-dramas: he produced a version of *Oedipus*, based on Yeats's play; a version of the *Bacchae* of Euripides; numerous other satyr-plays (after the Roman genre); and finally, a piece in Japanese Nôh-drama format, *Delusion of the Fury* (1968). To achieve his ends, Partch adapted and built new instruments, returning to the Just Intonation tuning-system of the Greeks, and using a 43-tone scale, *not* for mathematical reasons, but because only thus could instrumental music come really close to the microtonal expressive inflections of human speech. The power of vocalization, for Partch, is a 'bottle of cosmic vintage' which we are fools to reject. That power could be given also to instruments. All his instruments are based on Greek or oriental models – plectra, percussion instruments mainly, along with adapted viola, reed-organs and other accessories – and these are constructed with sufficient visual appeal to become the stage-sets (and even characters) in Partch's dramatic performances. The musicians are in costume, and take roles in the drama. Partch's music-theatre is thus highly integrated, but above all seeks a close bond with its audience through the insistence on a fundamental derivation of the music from vocal inflections.

Partch's attack on the abstract tradition of concert-music goes very deep. Its tenets are shaped by innumerable younger figures in the American and European avant-garde, who have sought to replace such a conception with a variety of theatrical presentations, investigating new links between performers, instruments and audience. The work of Larry Austin, Pauline Oliveros, David Reck and others in America, of Mauricio Kagel in Germany, Sylvano Bussotti in Italy, all harness a variety of musical media and techniques towards the discovery of alternatives to the European concert tradition.

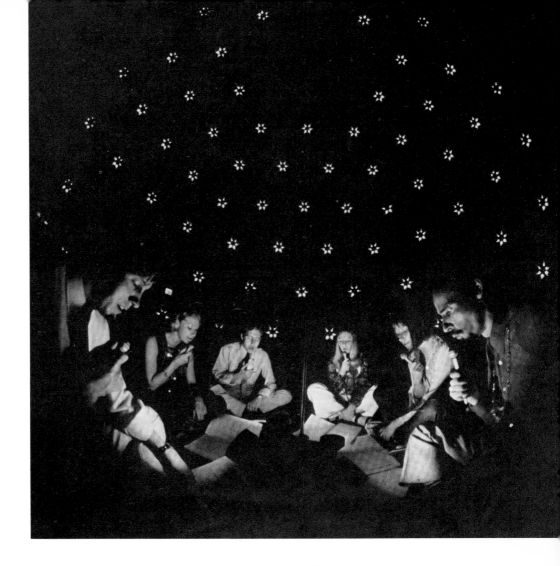

Some figures, such as Stockhausen, have moved from early preoccupation with post-Webern serialism towards a middle ground between the abstract and the corporeal: in Stockhausen's case, composer and audience meet in communal meditation – as in *Stimmung* (1968) and *Mantra* (1970), the former, incidentally, deriving entirely from vocalized sounds. Composers as apparently extreme in their support for abstraction in music as Babbitt, Xenakis and Lejaren Hiller (the last two are protagonists in computer composition) have all made concessions in the form of theatrical presentation that mediates between music and audience. Others, like Terry Riley, Steve Reich and Philip Glass, have explored links between systemic theory and 'phasing' processes in ethnic music (e.g. African drumming). With these, we have a return to a kind of simplicity that almost pre-supposes a 'popular' extension of their techniques such as we find in Mike Oldfield's *Tubular Bells*. Luciano Berio's preoccupation with linguistics, on the face of it an abstract concern, pure but not simple, boils down ultimately to a fascination with the expressive potential of vocalized sounds – their shaping by unconscious forces, especially taking into account the new pressure upon individuals within a mechanized world.

Composers, indeed, have been aware from the start of the century that machines can destroy feeling, yet they have been equally aware that new technological means can be utilized to give back to music many of the dimensions which it seemed to have lost within the prevailing modes of abstraction. Right from the provocative activities of the Italian futurists, in the first couple of decades of this century, an attack was clearly building up upon the exclusiveness and esoteric nature of the separately practised arts. Luigi Russolo, with his bizarre *intonarumori* (or noise-makers), welcomed the age of the automobile and factory-machines with open arms. Various Dadaists advocated the extension of musical language to include everyday noise. Most systematically, Edgard Varèse (1883–1965) saw his task as the 'liberation of sound', unshackled by the tempered system of tuning, traditional tonality and instrumental resources. He wrote his *Ionisation* (1932) for percussion ensemble with two sirens, introducing to Europe and America an entirely fresh sound-world. He advocated the use of electronic resources in composition in the 1920s, but was only able to acquire sufficiently dependable equipment to exploit electronic ideas in his compositions during the 1950s.

Varèse thought of music as spatial, as a phenomenon that moved in space. His *Poème électronique* (1958), conceived for and projected at the Philips Pavilion of the Brussels Exposition, made use of 400 loudspeakers carefully placed along the hyperbolic and parabolic curves of the structure designed by Le Corbusier, causing the sound to sweep in continuous arcs throughout the available space. In this respect, Varèse was aiming to revive concepts of musical experience that had been all but lost during the centuries in which musical abstraction had come to be dominant in the West.

In the church music of sixteenth- and seventeenth-century composers, for instance, this spacial facet had been fundamental. The sound moves around the listeners in the reverberant acoustic of churches and cathedrals, breaking through any tendency towards separateness or abstraction. The Gabrielis, Monteverdi, Cavalli and others all exploited this to an enormous extent, making the listener aware of many levels of play between foreground and background, an effect ensured by the planned distancing of the musical ingredients. Something of the same effect survived later in the music of both Berlioz and Bruckner. In Bruckner's symphonies, every key-change seems midwife to a modulation in distance, depth and perspective.

For a period, musicians attached much less importance to the spatial aspect of music. Now, in the modern epoch, electronics has supplied an infinitely flexible means for redressing the balance – given a new-found urge towards enveloping the listener in sound, as happens in many pop contexts. The ultimate may well be attained with the advancement of techniques in sonoholography, enabling the composer or performer to place and manipulate sounds in space in the most precise fashion. Taken together with holography, which can ultimately enable real, three-dimensional images to be placed, manipulated and moved around in space, the most spectacular forms of music-theatre might well be on the horizon.

Meanwhile, such technologies as exist have suggested to composers a whole range of subtle possibilities, whose influence is evident as much outside the electronic sphere as within it. For instance, composers now make great play with structures depending upon variation of focus. In Stockhausen's *Gesang der Jünglinge* (a tape-composition dating from 1958), for instance, the music is perceived on several levels: one where vocal sounds are heard with total clarity; a blurred level, where the strands and detailed components are half-perceived; and a pure noise level, where no coherence is to be found. Its interest and fascination subsist in the interplay between such levels. Such a notion has been developed in diverse forms, using only live performers: e.g. Ligeti, in his *Chamber Concerto* (1969) and many other pieces; and Berio, in his *Sinfonia* (1968). With Ligeti the effect is not unlike that of Op Art: it is a play upon the aural perceptions. With Berio, it amounts to a probing inside the human psyche, wherein familiar quotations, nightmare distortions and blurred transformations are always mixed together. Berio, inspired by Joyce, deliberately applies a 'stream of consciousness' method, something familiar in film and literature from early in the century, but new to music.

In today's music, therefore, it is apparently possible for music to incorporate many feelings or none. It has been demoted to the status of background – soothing or stimulating, in airport lounge or factory floor – by the Muzak company. The range of possibilities is so great that a figure like John Cage would say that the choice of what can be regarded as music and what cannot should be allowed entirely to the listener; the composer must abdicate from his position of tyrannical authority, and at best can demonstrate the indeterminate nature of creative enterprise. The implications of specific choices, made by those who do not take the Cage line – the majority – are not easy to define. In the rock sphere, the furthest possibility is of a change of life-style. Feelings are here associated with an anarchist outlook. Outside this sphere, the artist seems in general to be continuing an age-old process whereby he serves his own and his brothers' and sisters' inner needs. The 'feeling' with which he is dealing is a marriage of many impulses, desires, hopes and ambitions, a drive towards perceptual adventure, a yearning for security and stability, for integrity and wholeness. The polarities and self-contradictions are manifold. Thus the artist has *many* roles – and there is room for both the abstract and the corporeal.

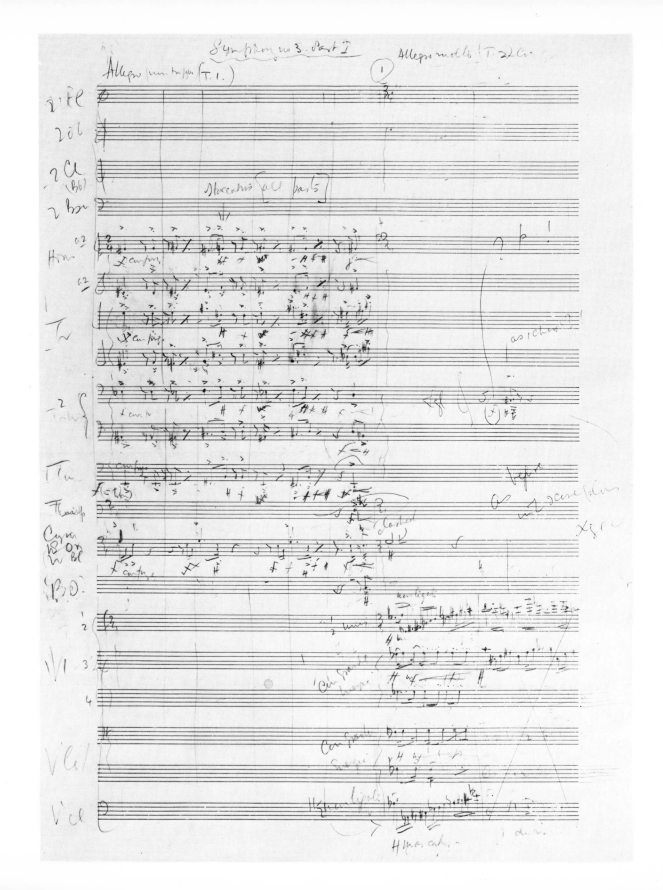

MICHAEL TIPPETT

Sir Michael Tippett is one of our greatest living composers. Since his war-time oratorio, *A Child of our Times*, his creative output has won him international recognition. He has composed three symphonies and four major operas: *The Midsummer Marriage, King Priam, The Knot Garden*, and *The Ice Break*.

Tippett's original pencil draft of the opening of his Third Symphony.

Feelings of inner experience

You may wonder what link exists between the work of the creative artist at this time and the very common present pursuit of sensation, the desire to make more out of our feelings and senses. I think it's possible we've moved into a world in which all of us, young and old, want to develop a feeling in our bodies that in some way counterbalances the extreme boredom, mechanization and soullessness of a great deal of our life. This is an exaggerated way of putting it. Yet why this tremendous increase in the demand for music over the whole world? Young people play music to an extent that never happened before. I have a feeling that this is going to be signally of our epoch. I imagine this period now is one in which everybody wants to come closer to this experience within themselves – to play, to dream, to have these interior notions which can only be obtained through sounds, through visual things, through dancing – and also, I suppose, through hallucinatory drugs: for a hallucinatory drug will take you into a visionary world.

An artist like myself, who doesn't need to take drugs to enter a visionary world – and who is in a way hostile to the idea of such willed stimulus – has but to reach out with his 'metaphorical hand', and put the music down, because this music comes by instinct, a re-awakening inside the physical body, so that the stomach perhaps moves as the music moves. The movements of the stomach or any other part of the nervous system, in response to the *imagined* music, is the somatic test of aesthetic validity within the combined psycho-somatic act of creation – just as sets of gradually acquired intellectual judgments of formal patternings, of taste, of values, are the tests of the conscious mind. When the music thus imagined is performed the process in the listener may be reversed – a psycho-somatic response may be engendered that is analogous, or even similar, to the finally accepted optimum of the composer's tests. To *some* degree, the more primitive, unsophisticated, the music in question, the more the somatic dominates the psychic. The listener's body in fact may seemingly be forced into actual movement. I've watched this happen in the heart of the African bush, with people dancing and jiving (to the same kind of vernacular music we know in Europe or America) until they themselves are receptive to some kind of totally absorbing interior emotion. Now that is a long way from sitting in the Royal Festival Hall, London, to listen to a piece of composed, sophisticated music; but it's not so long that the thing isn't in some essential way joined. This is, as it were, the ground upon which I must put my feet when I write.

173

216

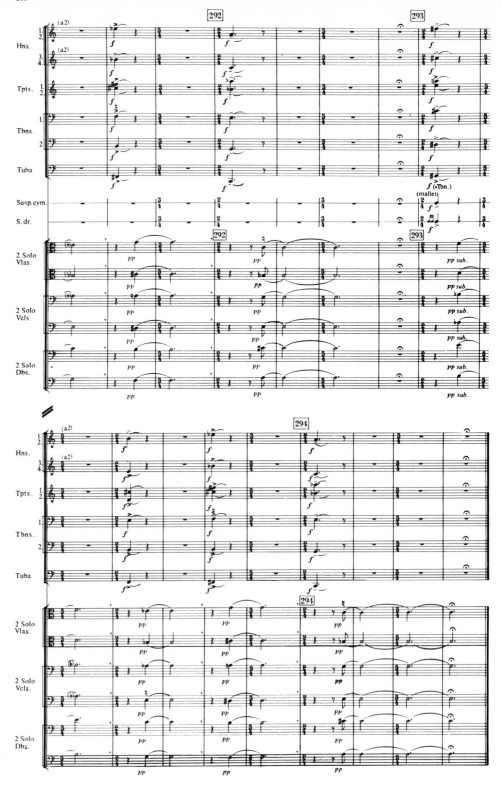

When I ask myself what music does really express, I find it difficult to define in words: not because words are another medium (for words, apart from their use in poetry, are the proper medium for definition), but because there is here something of the indefinable. However, there are certain things I *can* tell you about it. For instance, it must be concerned with the interior of my psyche – a very difficult term, because I don't even know where the psyche is, in the body or in the mind. But this is the vital thing. It's not about the sensations apprehended from the external world, but about the intimations, intuitions, dreams, fantasies, emotions, the feelings within ourselves. Insofar as poets use words and others use materials from the external world to express these feelings, I use sound. Whatever happens in the outside world – and I do take from the outside world – it must be in some way transmuted. Now this is a magical process which I cannot describe accurately. Nobody, indeed, knows what it is. And yet I have to operate it. Moreover, I operate it from a necessity so strong that I have only gradually come to accept it openly, and to understand that this obsessive process continues, persists, and may be so strong that I'm mystified finally as to what was in the outside world.

I've learnt, of course, that if I went too far and allowed the whole of my external ordinary experience to be dominated by this transmutatory process, then I should go mad – it would be like schizophrenia. You have, as an artist, a very delicate balance between matter-of-factness and allowing – again I must use a complicated bodily metaphor – something inside to tremble, some membrane to vibrate, which enables the unconscious (whatever that is), the intimations, dreams to come through a kind of gateway into an apprehendable form. For as soon as this happens, I have to use rational processes upon it – my sense of shape or form. I have to polarize these two, the irrational psychic instructions and the rational formality, in some such way that it's set down finally as a collection of notes and instructions for music. Not that I get an emotion from this set of notes and instructions, but if they are heard in the concert hall, something of this strange transmutatory magical experience happens to you from the sounds you physically hear. If the work finally is a good one you would go absolutely and entirely with it. Why we want this nobody knows, but human beings certainly do need it as part of something for which I think we must use the word Soul. We want our souls to be nourished, and unless they are, we are dead.

When I am composing, the mundane, external world distracts me violently. When I am so lost in the process of playing, say, trying to find the music I need, perhaps playing everything so softly it's almost impossible to hear, if somebody comes into the room, or the telephone rings, the shock is sharp. I've got used to it, I can deal with it, but this only means that the external world is annoying during the process of creation. On the other hand, I would be an absolutely non-existent human being if I hadn't been moved by a bird's song, by music, by the sound of water, of trees: not only the sounds of nature, but the sounds of somebody playing on a trumpet, the sounds of pop music coming through the window – all these things are stored up in the mind.

If that condition of mind and soul, which we call inspiration, *lasted long without intermission, no artist could survive it. The strings would break and the instrument be shattered into fragments.*
Peter Ilyich Tchaikovsky

Closing bars of the Third Symphony (printed score).

175

If you look at the printed score of my *Third Symphony* you see it is a finished entity. It has many pages; it has thousands, perhaps millions, of notes. Now those notes have been invented by me as a series of instructions for people to be able to perform the work. I have in principle nothing to do with the performance: my concern is simply with invention. The invention must of course be such that the instructions are accurate, precise to the last possible detail – though the last detail is not totally possible. That's how far we go.

Now all that takes a very great deal of time and energy to create. You have a process whereby something begins – and the beginning is the strangest part of it, because it is spontaneous. In this case, for instance, I can tell you exactly how it happened. I was in a concert at the Edinburgh Festival once when there was a piece of modern music being played – much of it very slow, almost immobile. I found myself saying that if ever I wanted to use that kind of music I would have to match it with something extremely sharp, violent, and certainly speedy. In retrospect, I realize that I had gone from the sounds coming to my ears from the outside world, in which a concert was being played, to the interior world inside my own body. In my own mind the process of invention was beginning. I didn't go very far. I recall merely saying to my neighbour, 'The *Third Symphony* has begun!'

The work took seven years of intermittent consideration and eventual creation. From such tiny noting of a future possibility I had to put down a kind of mnemonic shorthand, so that I could remember what I thought the structure of the whole work might be when I'd only experienced the initial moment of conception. Plate (3) reproduces one of the mnemonics for the *Third Symphony* where a great many disjointed, unstructured notions have been noted in my own kind of verbal shorthand. There you can see simple statements about all the possibilities that there might be in the symphony. Some will be discarded, some kept. But the original spontaneous conception of 'immobile' polarized against 'speedy' (so ridiculously simple, but clearly having the power to initiate the creative process now apparently ready to begin) was always the structuring factor.

While holding these ideas in my mind over a period of years, allowing them gradually to grow, I come next to a moment when I had nearly everything in my mind except the notes. The symphony so far had a structure and balance; it had ideas about orchestration. Thus I could begin what is usually thought of as the composition. I began at the piano a search for the right sounds. Now I don't find the precise sounds I want *on* the piano, but *through* the piano (this is after all a piece for an orchestra). But I can invent *as though* the orchestral score were in my head all the time. When I tried to find the sharp chords for the start (I even thought they were something like an engine waiting to burst into action) it was only guesswork, as I had to search for such sounds over and over again. When I had got them absolutely dead clear, then I wrote them down. On a faded piece of paper (p. 172) are almost one hundred per cent accurate indications as to what those chords are made of – sounds for trumpets, trombone, horns; rhythms for percussion. It's just possible to

With clarity and quiet, I look upon the world and say:

All that I see, hear, taste, smell, and touch are the creations of my mind.

The sun comes up and the sun goes down in my skull.

Out of one of my temples the sun rises, and into the other the sun sets.

The stars shine in my brain; ideas, men, animals browse in my temporal head; songs and weeping fill the twisted shells of my ears and storm the air for a moment.

My brain blots out, and all, the heavens and the earth, vanish.

The mind shouts: 'Only I exist!'

Deep in my subterranean cells my five senses labour; they weave and unweave space and time, joy and sorrow, matter and spirit.
Nikos Kazantzakis

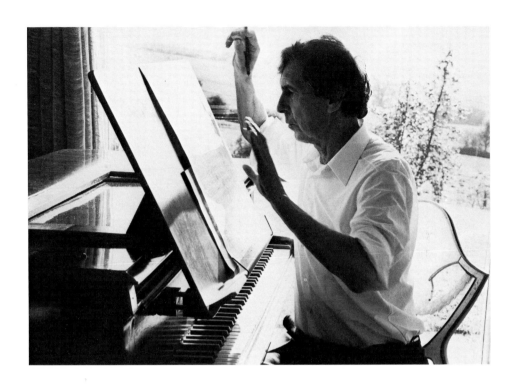

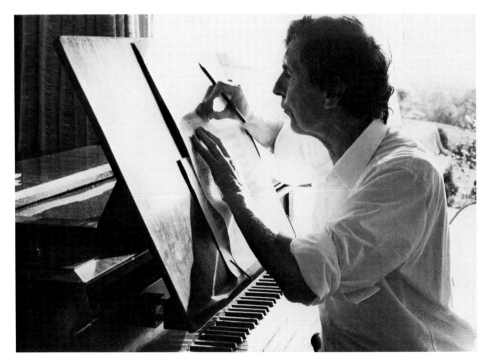

Sir Michael Tippett.

see on the end of the page a lot of fast notes for strings and woodwind, when the music has exploded into the air. So there you have the original germinal, but soundless, idea actualized into written notes. On page 174 is the very end of the symphony, where the germ has become 'tough' versus 'tender' in some metaphor of acceptance.

I think everyone has to a certain extent the capacity to express this inner world, but it varies in degree. Nearly all children have this ability. Instinctively, a child would take a crayon – even if he was going eventually to be a musician – for it's much easier to put what you imagine down like that with your hand on the crayon. The techniques of music are much more complicated. It's only lately that we are beginning to understand that the child might accomplish musical work if he played with his toys to make sounds from them. We haven't got quite that far yet. But the thing that is going to make children in later life into real poets, painters, composers, architects, sculptors is a gift; a special gift, no doubt: it is the obsessional quality – I can't put it better than that.

Force lines of the psycho-magnetic field surrounding the human head. From S. Babbit, *Principles of Light and Colour.*

PERSONAL POTENTIAL:
transforming your experience

Concentration is the key. In 'normal' states of mind our conscious energies are scattered. Our attention wanders aimlessly from thought to thought, to external sensations to internal sensations, to the past, to the future, to snatches of tunes, to hopes and fears, to images and objects. Nearly all systems of meditation require preliminary practice at concentration, at stilling the restlessness of the ever-observing mind. Meditation is nothing more than directed concentration. Concentration is power.

Andrew Weil

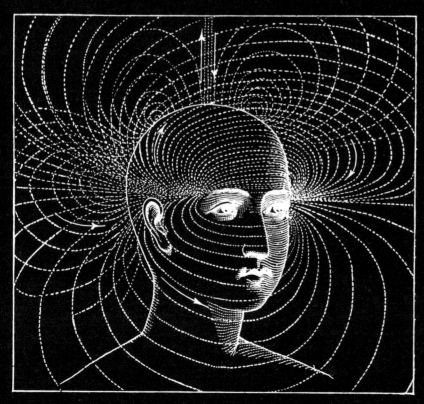

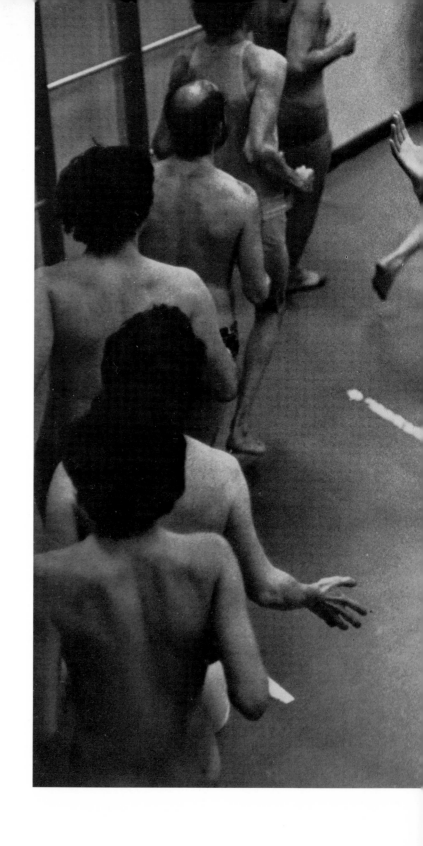

A bioenergetic workshop.

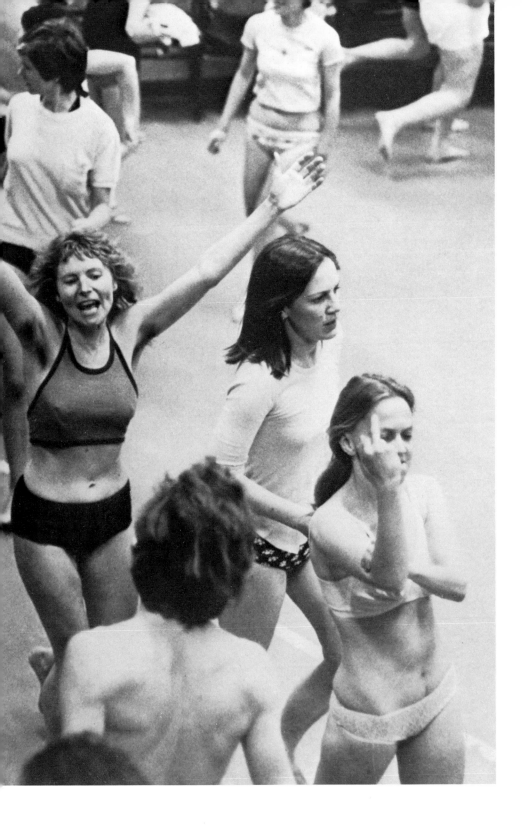

People will do anything, no matter how absurd, in order to avoid facing their own souls. They will practise Indian yoga and all its exercises, observe a strict regime of diet, learn the literature of the whole world – all because they cannot get on with themselves and have not the slightest faith that anything useful could ever come out of their own souls. Thus the soul has gradually been turned into a Nazareth from which nothing good can come. Therefore let us fetch it from the four corners of the earth – the more far fetched and bizarre it is the better.

C. G. Jung

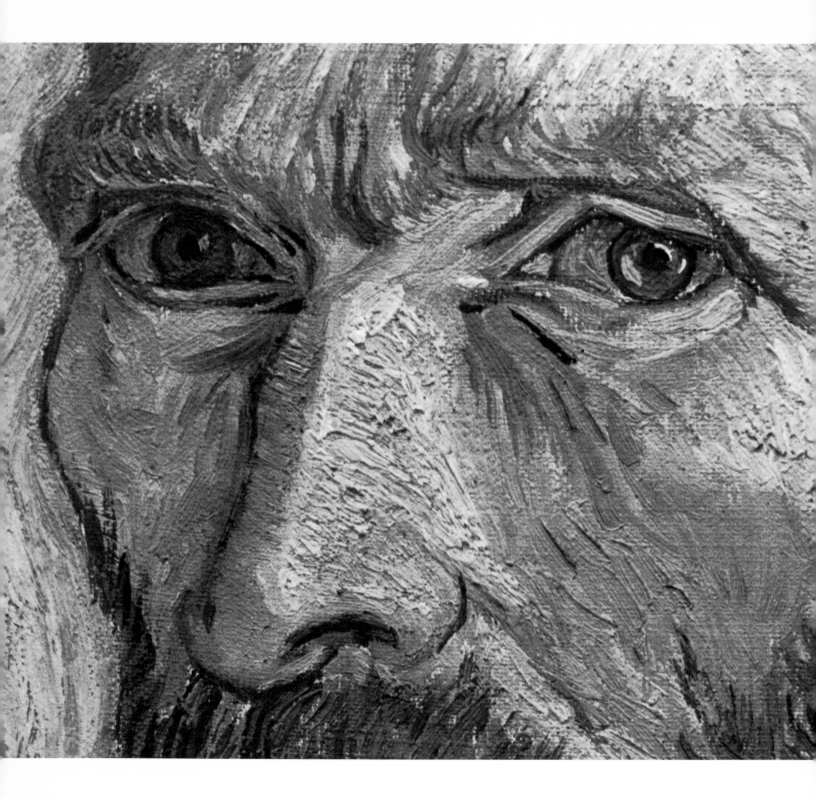

Light out of darkness

BANI SHORTER

The experience of Jungian analysis

Bani Shorter works as a Jungian analyst in London. Here she outlines the process of self-discovery which underlines many of the activities described in the chapters that follow.

Dusk to dawn, chrysalis to moth, cave to resurrection – all these are symbols of becoming; by way of darkness, towards light. Since time immemorial and in all places people have used these symbols to describe the enclosure, loneliness, eventual release and renewal of a transforming experience. Darkness is synonymous with death and unknowing; light with birth and recognition. The kindling of fire signifies the return of both light and warmth, as exemplified by the lighting of candles on the Christmas tree at the darkest and coldest season of the year. Likewise, the single candle symbolizes the unique and glowing potential of an individual life.

In his autobiography, C. G. Jung, the founder of analytical psychology, relates a dream in which he carries a tiny light that threatens to go out at any moment. This imagery suggests an experience familiar to all of us. We take our journeys through life trying to protect our individual flames from extinction. What threatens them may be the winds of society's opinion, our own carelessness, in some instances ambition, neglect or our leaving them in the care of others. But if the flame dies out, the world becomes a dark and frightening place. We lose both our way and the one way to find a way. In this regard, we are all familiar with the gaunt and listless faces of those who have been imprisoned or the victims of concentration camps, pictures whose withered forms remain to haunt us. Yet at the same time we can be quite callous to our inner prisoners, long constrained and tortured memories asking for attention and release.

Light, the kindling of light, and the return of light are associated with analysis, both by way of symbolism and analogy. When we analyse we re-enact the pattern and symbolism of all growth: darkness, descent, withering and winter giving way to dawn, ascent, sprouting and spring. Analysis is not a form; it is a natural psychological process involving both upper and lower, light and dark, the conscious and unconscious sides of the personality in new relationship and, eventually, synthesis.

The story of one's becoming a more nearly complete and at the same time a more singular person often begins with the words, 'I know there's no logical reason for it to happen, and yet . . .' This seems an irrational summons, and to the person familiar with conscious, intellectualized existence, the impact of such a message is startling. While it may not be unusual to feel one has reached the limit of one's energy and

Detail from a Van Gogh self-portrait, 1889–90.

resources for good reasons, it is another matter to reach an impasse contrary to the logic of outer circumstance. Nothing works, at least not according to established and manageable routines. One has a sense of losing control or, worse, of being in the hands of a perverse fate. One no longer feels in possession of one's own soul. Worse even than the thoughts of suicide which may accompany such a state is the feeling of death-in-life.

Initially, those who come into analysis experience despair and a dark night of the soul. Analysis brings relief with insight and awareness of what may have caused the pent-up anger, frustration or despair. But superficial answers do not suffice. They seldom satisfy and do not heal. Inwardly, this search involves retreat, waiting and transformation.

I have watched children close their eyes to play at being blind and I have observed blind children try to orient themselves to a seeing world. The experience of watching the neurotic sufferer is different, however. Not only is he deprived of light but he can no longer believe light exists. He has lost his hold on life. He may have lost his job, his health or his family. Hope and purpose have been eclipsed. He lives in shadow, at least in part; and by way of analysis we must recover the lost sun, representing his energy, his consciousness and creative strength. We take our cues not from an outer world prescribed by predictable and recognizable patterns, but search for cues in the inner world, beyond the realm of light and sight. The healing images form in the inner, vague and unpredictable recesses of the personality which is both individual and collective, old and ever-new, lustrous and sordid, as well as the storehouse of all that is repressed, rejected, or reprehensible to the outer personality.

This remote and hidden side of ourselves is called the unconscious. Of the many worlds which humans inhabit simultaneously, the one most neglected until recently was this, the world within. Not until the end of the last century did Freud, then Jung and others, begin to explore and describe this dark region in its own terms. Since then, depth psychologists have been engaged in a continual search for the meaning of the fantastic images and enigmatic symbols cast up by it, while individual therapy has been directed toward the integration of these meanings into life.

The process of discovery and integration of the hitherto unseen and unacknowledged parts of the personality is what goes on in a Jungian analysis, conducted, in Jungian terms, 'one to one and face to face'. But the dynamic and moving force is always the presence of need, or temporary imbalance; that is, psychological suffering and disturbance. On the ego or performance level the need may be described as an inability to achieve, risk or perform. At another level, however, called the level of the self, the disturbance may be felt as a longing of the soul for expression and meaning. The redress of the balance between inner longing and outer performance is the goal of the work and results in something closer to a totality of personality. To achieve this end analyst and analysand set forth on a journey into the unknown. The course of observing the continuities of inner happenings by way of fantasies, dreams and synchronicities is unique. Over time

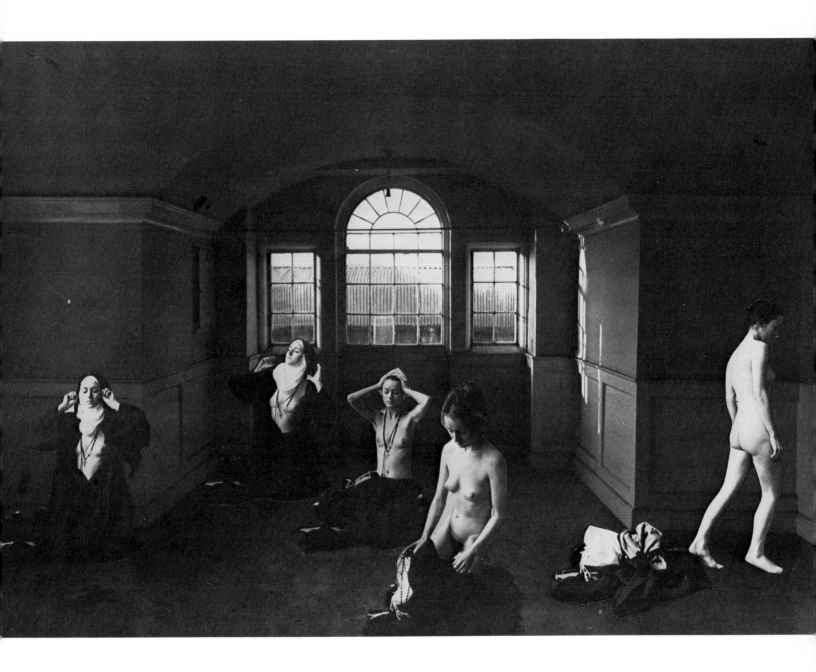

Photomontage from *An Exorcism* by Penny
Slinger.

and with the strengthening of the conscious personality what happens amounts to the unfolding of an individual myth.

Analysis is not an intellectual search; it is a therapeutic one, undertaken out of necessity, to recover a sense of proportion, balance or control. In the presence of the experienced therapist, it is an awesome and numinous but nonetheless an exacting task. It deals with vagaries but it is not itself vague. The language of symbolism which speaks through the dreams, the nightmares, and the fantasies is unerringly precise and demanding, designed as it is for the living of the one unique, individual life. Development in the direction of realizing one's deepest self is a highly personal undertaking. In fact, because of its specific and individual nature, an analysis cannot be discussed in categorical terms but only by way of mythic parallels. The same type of dream may be dreamed by more than one person but the one dream is not repeated. That is the dreamer's own.

By way of illustration of the kind of threshold phenomenon which can startle a person at a crossroads of decision, setting a new direction and conveying a sense of other-worldly intervention, is the following dream, reported by a woman in her early fifties:

> I was back in the city where I was born and lived as a child. I was walking in a formal park or sculpture garden. I was attracted by the many statues which had been sculpted in the style of my youth. As I strolled among them I became aware that they wanted me to do something for them. They wanted me to feed them. In a nest of shrubbery I came upon a statue of myself aged nine. I stopped to look at it. When I did, it reached out its arms of stone and with a soundless voice begged for nourishment.

The image of being turned to stone is apt. It occurs again and again. At the outset of analysis rigidity is expressed in many forms. 'I've become locked into a routine,' one person says, speaking of why he has sought the help of an analyst. 'I can no longer get myself to work,' admits someone else. 'I feel as if I were carrying the weight of the world,' another says; 'If only I could cry.' For many, time has slowed almost to a halt. It seems pointless to plan a meal, to go to a party, to take a holiday. No one can think where to go; there is no longer any place where he wants to go. He stares out of the window and is aware of that most barren of all feelings, the feeling of having no feeling. There is a freezing over of the personality, a loss of sensitivity and a coldness akin to the onset of death.

Here we have the familiar fairy-tale motif of the spirit locked in stone, confined in a bottle, or enclosed in a glass coffin. The dreamer who met herself as a child and a statue said, 'When I dreamed that, I felt as if I were in a fairy-tale.' Without her seeking it, in the midst of a life which demanded a multitude of family, social and professional commitments she received this surprising summons. She had neither requested nor planned for the dream. Instead, it appeared to have been delivered from a remote, transpersonal centre of her being beyond rational control. She

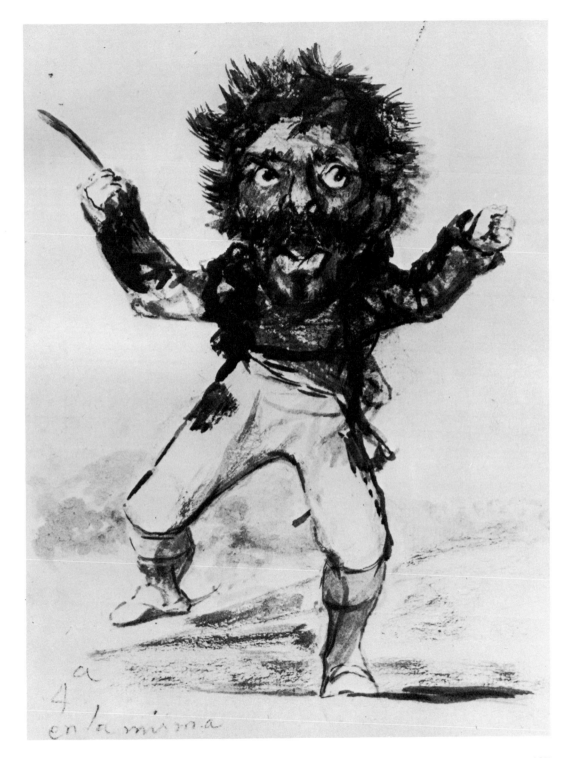

Goya, *The Nightmare.*

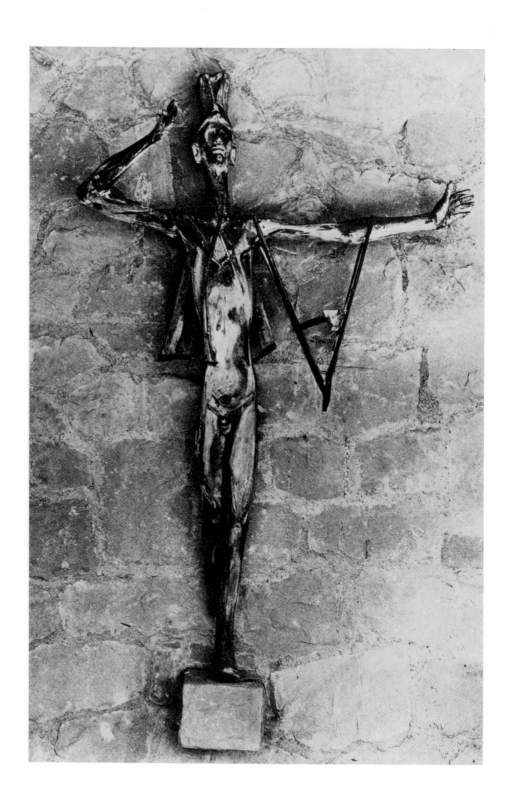

Emilio Stanzani's statue *The Dreamseller.*

herself, that is, the waking ego, was given only the choice of ignoring or acknowledging its message.

Dreams and other communications from the unconscious which may come in the form of fantasies, synchronicities, or even spontaneous pictures and visions are accompanied by a sense of remoteness, other-worldliness and numinosity which makes them hard to forget. They want to be taken seriously. This, combined with their personal relevance, eventually forces the analysand to confront the possibility of an irrational but valid centre in himself from which such messages arise. At first what is communicated from this 'other' personality may appear to be dispassionate and disconnected from the life the individual is living. Only later does he realize that, taken in sequence, such messages express a bias, a bias on the side of his becoming more completely what he alone can be.

A compensatory process is at work. All that the individual may be but is not yet is reflected in his unconscious life, which acts like a mirror to his everyday and conscious strivings. Recognizing this, if a person then takes it into account, he finds renewed energy at his disposal and he is able to recover a sense of well-being. If, however, he ignores the help offered by his unconscious, he seems to go against his destiny and promise. The curious existence of an inner regulatory voice gives the impression of another and more objective presence. Jung himself referred to it as the presence of the objective psyche or a manifestation of the archetype of the self.

At the point in an analysis when the analysand accepts the possibility of a compensatory wisdom hidden in the dark core of his being there is a danger he will let go conscious controls. The situation is made all the more acute by the magnetic fascination of the archetypal images he encounters, the most numinous of which is the archetype of the self, synonymous with the god within. There is a danger of giving way to its seductive enchantment – like Merlin, of falling under a spell, surrendering to its power. Giddy with the possibilities of expanded consciousness, an inflated ego prepares to revel in a feast of unexpected and other-worldly delights.

When, however, this critical point is reached and there is the temptation of the ego's over-reaching itself, when there is a danger of analysis becoming not a process but an end or a substitute, one of several things may happen. Most likely is the receipt of a summons to return to the realities of day-to-day living. In whatever symbolism it is couched, the summons acts like a letter delivered to a person in a faraway place, recalling him to a sense of his identity and vocation. Though arising from the unconscious, its fulfilment will demand conscious co-operation. Expressed in the difficult language of symbols, its meaning may not be evident immediately. But in the process of decoding, that is to say, in the interaction between outer life and its inner referrant, a different and stronger personality comes into being, an ego is formed which incorporates and fulfils more of its unique potential. A new totality is formed.

At this juncture such a message was received by a young artist. It came in the form of a dream. He was a person who had turned his back on a career for which he was particularly well suited and had decided to give himself to what he felt were more socially relevant and appealing pursuits. These concerns were beguiling for him, and he became infatuated with a rather one-sided way of life. Being the opposite of that for which he was best fitted, these interests seduced him further and further from his natural calling and seemed at times to be encouraged by both his conscious and unconscious. At the point of greatest fascination and activity, however, he dreamed:

> I was travelling from east to west and had come to a desert. I was alone and thirsty. Suddenly, from behind me, I heard the sound of approaching footsteps. An old man was running to catch up with me. He had travelled a long way to bring me a package which contained my brushes and paint.

The exploration of one of these dreams and its interpretation is sobering. Such a highly personal communication will have an impact far stronger than any moral or academic injunction to return to work, rising as it does from the depths of one's own being and bringing with it an authority backed by strength and encouraging confidence. Answering it, a person has a sense of coming into the inheritance of what is rightfully his, the chance to develop and live out his natural gifts. Inner and outer possibilities recombine in a new pattern.

If the return journey of an analysis can be charted it begins with that discovery of who one is and must be, not in mature form but in embryo, as it were. This is the start of the process called 'individuation'. Here the light is rekindled. It is an experience paralleled in the death and rebirth symbolism of all initiation ceremonies.

Moments of breakthrough which come at such times are profoundly moving. When the spirit imprisoned in stone is finally freed, the throb and pulse of life return. Transformation becomes more than a concept; it is an evident release of feeling, sensation, and purpose which shows itself in living terms. The analysand no longer assumes a mask; he inherits his face. In the same way, he reclaims and inhabits his body. Others often remark, 'He seems so much more himself all of a sudden.' Both analyst and analysand know it has not happened all of a sudden. It is the result of long, patient work and waiting. But every time it does happen – that some hitherto unconscious part of the personality is regained – there is a sense of letting go, redefining a border, shedding an out-worn cloak, renewal.

Little by little the one who felt himself to be cut off and estranged learns to trust a different part of himself which is available to guide and support his life's decisions and activities. Consequently, the analyst becomes less important as support, guide, or interpreter; for as the direction of the individual journey becomes clearer, the person's own ability to take his journey develops. Not all messages from the unconscious are of equal depth or value but over time they can be seen to circle round a central core of possibilities which is both limited and boundless. These are the possibilities of becoming what one is. Those who are able to establish a dialogue with these possibilities move between conscious and unconscious life in ceaseless

Der Traum ('The Dream') – painting by one of Bani Shorter's patients.

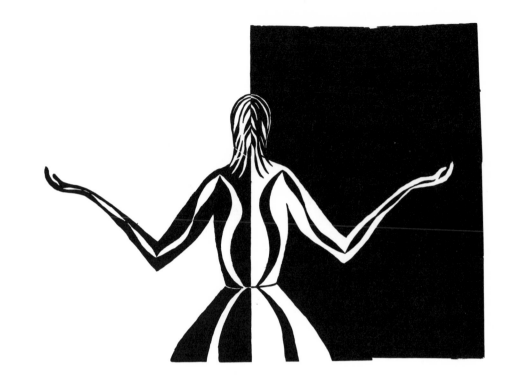

'She worships the wall,' said the patient.

Spiral. Both these paintings are by Bani Shorter's patients.

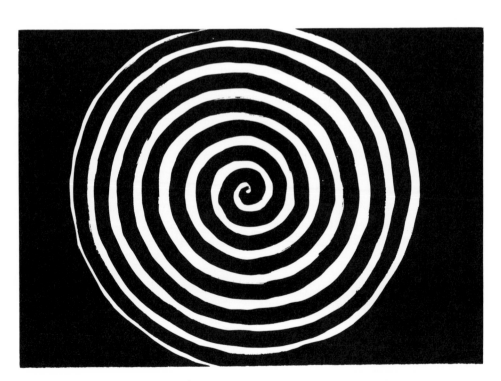

alternation on a path which links the deepest darkness of unknowing with the light of awareness.

'I dreamed I was in a small house of my own,' reported a woman in her sixties who for most of her years lived a life in conformity with the aspirations of others. This precipitated a major crisis which brought her into analysis. Here she began to discover the possibility of having space for the expression of her own personality. 'The house was built of stone covered by mud or plaster,' she continued:

> The walls had been fashioned and smoothed by hand. There were three rooms in this house; mine was the middle room but there was a room above and one below. Between the rooms were openings. It was as if I could be seen by whoever occupied the other rooms and I myself could move back and forth between them. I don't remember there being any windows in this house but there must have been, for the place was filled with light.

The dream poetically describes the appropriate position of a conscious ego which functions independently but has access to all that may be symbolized by the lower and higher parts of the personality: ignorance and awareness, the life of the body and the reality of the spirit, that which signifies deepest darkness and transcendence. Between the opposites is a light-filled space prepared to be inhabited by the individual.

Along the path of individual development explored in analysis and called individuation, the symbol stands as beacon and marker. Its indiscernible but numinous beckoning rouses one again and again to consider the way, both how and for what purposes it is taken. For the symbol is not absolute. It is relevant to time, circumstance and the receiver. Sometimes no more than the bare outlines of its meaning can be seen by historic references – such parallels, for example, may say nothing about the individual context. There are also hazards connected with being too quick to interpret, too literal, too exact. It is only by attentive and appreciative application that one can coax forth the hidden content of a symbol. And when one does, it is so often other than one had assumed. Yet only when that happens can it take its place, rather like one of a series of lamps lighting the way along a dark tunnel.

The time a person spends in analysis is sometimes long and often difficult. We go into darkness and explore it not for its own sake but for the sake of what is waiting there for us. ' . . . he would have us remember most of all to be enthusiastic over the night,' Auden wrote of the father of the analytic method:

> *not only for the sense of wonder*
> *it alone has to offer, but also*
> *because it needs our love. With large sad eyes*
> *its delectable creatures look up and beg*
> *us dumbly to ask them to follow:*
> *they are exiles who long for the future*
> *that lies in our power.*

We submit our way but we do not surrender to the unconscious; for if we were to surrender there would no longer be the possibility of dialogue. Nevertheless we learn to follow mysterious summonings which come from a centre of the personality beyond rational control and we value these summonings for their light- and life-giving potential, value them even when at times they illumine things we do not wish to see. As this happens, through a process of constant reflection upon the centre, slowly, out of the darknesss and ambiguity of unknowing, possibilities of transformation are revealed and integrated.

It is obvious that in this work the analysand goes a way others have gone before and will always go, as witnessed by the transformation rites and ceremonies of all peoples and recorded in their living dreams which come down to us in the form of myths and legends, fairy and folk-tales. Psychologically, the way involves meeting certain recognizable and familiar figures better identified as archetypes of the psyche; the shadow, the contrasexual companion, mana personalities such as the old man of the young artist's dream, and the self. Yet what the analysand himself experiences is more than a happening or a repetition of what others have discovered. The journey that he takes into the recesses of his psyche is not all journeys nor yet 'any' journey. It is distinctly personal. The light which he goes to seek and with which he returns from the encounter with darkness, pain and suffering is the light which illuminates the one life that is his own.

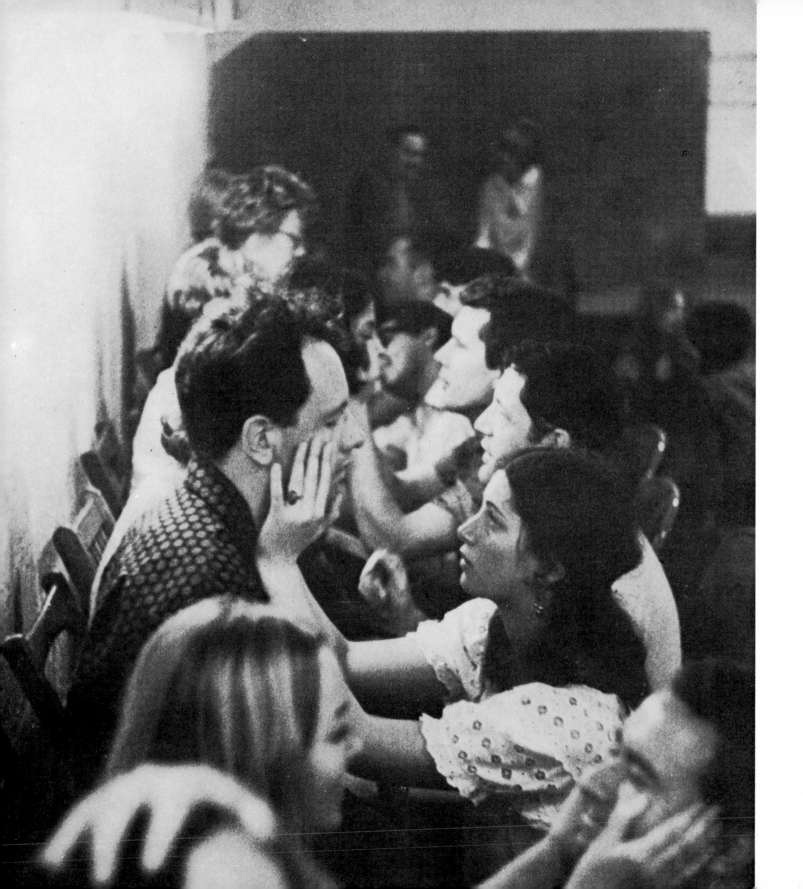

TOM FALKNER

Tom Falkner leads Encounter Groups all over Europe. In this chapter he describes an incident which was photographically recorded during an evening session. The group had already been together for five weekends and was then meeting regularly two nights every week. There was no agenda, only a process of interaction.

Encounter

In order that no movement be inhibited, the room's only furniture is cushions. We kneel, sit, sprawl, and frequently change positions. There is enough space for the whole group of fourteen people to do warm-up exercises or simply dance. Also the room is sound-proofed, so we can feel free to shout or even scream.

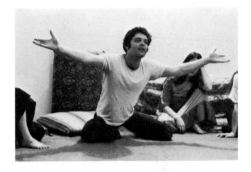

Sometimes I cause my role as leader to stop my own expression. I feel my chest constricted, my heart thumping. Letting go frees me from the restriction of having to be right.

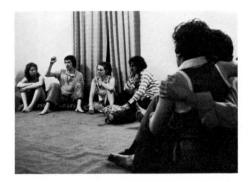

The focus of attention turned to Sacha, the man with his arm raised. He woke that morning suddenly recalling an incident in childhood – the sound of his father's voice in another room shouting at his mother.

195

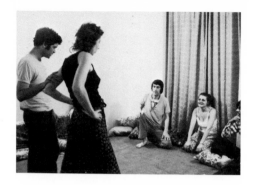

Sacha chose Joanna, who was sitting next to him, as his mother in the group and myself as father to re-create the original conflict. Before he chose the parental figures, both Joanna and I 'knew' we would be involved. This 'knowing' beforehand seems to suggest that something much deeper than a mere casting of parts has taken place. Something about Joanna and me and our relationship in the present evokes the same emotional response Sacha felt towards his parents. Rather than mere acting, our own authentic response is an essential part of the work which follows.

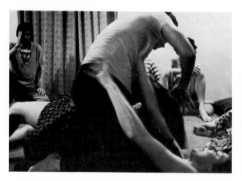
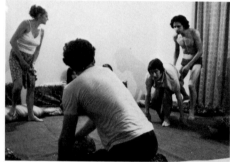

A visual structure based on action is much closer to real and primitive emotion than language. From the story it seemed Sacha feared that his father would hurt his mother. I wrestled Joanna to the floor. Sacha sat frozen, unable to move. Though I am holding Joanna down my attention is towards Sacha. This might be the clue that Sacha's real fear is his father's violence turning on him. Joanna withdrew from the action which followed. The conflict was to play itself out between father and son. Carole, the group's co-leader, and another group member encouraged Sacha to move forward to meet his father. In actual physical contact Sacha's emotional energy changed from fear to anger.

196

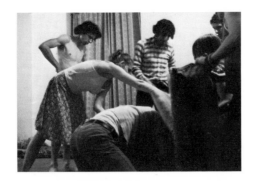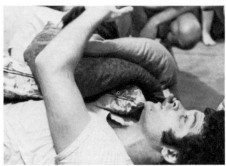

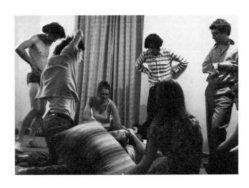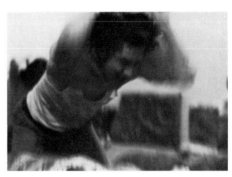

Carole stepped in to place a pillow on top of me, for protection. Then Sacha started to hit. His pent-up reaction to the threatening father broke loose. He was then in touch with his own violence. There were no words but he was yelling savagely. Perhaps buried in his unconscious was the primitive feeling of murder toward his father.

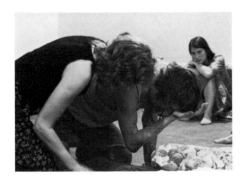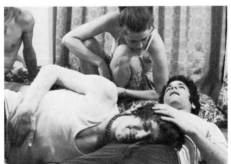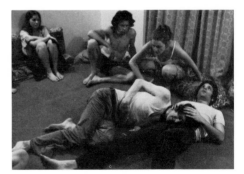

The violence spent, Sacha's feeling changed to guilt. Joanna moved in to confront him. I remember myself thinking, 'There is more between us – his interest is still with me – the father.' Sensing the same thing, Carole directed Sacha to put his head on my stomach. He began to cry in pain and remorse – the consequence of having felt and experienced the hatred towards a father for whom he has also felt love.

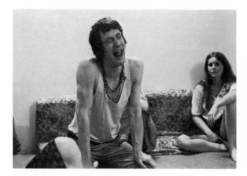 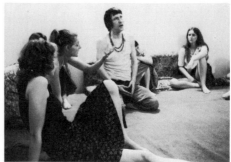

Carole intervened to set up a structure to finally unite Sacha and his father. Sacha was on his knees facing me. The structure was arranged so that he had to look up at me, as a young boy would look up at his father.

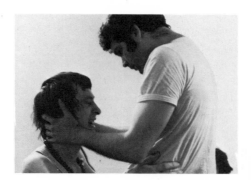

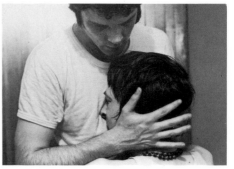

The next step was a symbolic declaration of the paternal and filial bond. I simply said, 'I am your father, you are my son.' Carole asked Sacha to repeat the words from his side. Far from interrupting the bond between us, Carole's outside instruction got right to the centre of Sacha's feeling. As he said, 'I am your son, you are my father', he felt fully the deep pain of longing to be united with his father.

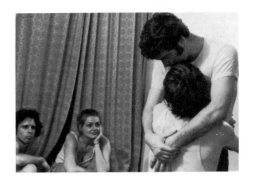

As we joined, I felt my own tenderness towards Sacha. His hands on my sides, at first shy and delicate, gave way to a strong embrace. His breathing became long heaving sighs. The frozen ambivalence of conflicting feelings had unwound itself in a natural sequence as each of us was allowed full expression. Sacha's deep sighs continued, and we remained clasped together for some time. The sighs spoke of rest and well-being. The events of childhood cannot be altered or relived. Yet throughout life remains the urge to express the uncompleted feelings. Sacha was still on his knees as a not fully-grown child.

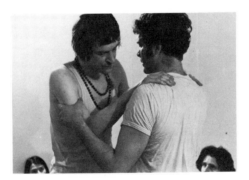

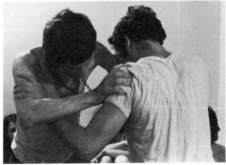

After the period of rest he rose to his feet. He felt older now and as his hands grasped my shoulders I felt my own hands on his biceps. Spontaneously our movement developed into a contest. As an adolescent feels and tests his strength, we locked together and pushed. At length Sacha succeeded in pushing me right back into a corner.

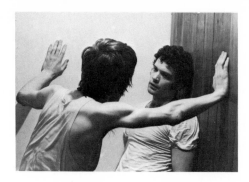

This moment marked the climax of my participation. I was tired and wanted to rest. I was wondering to what extent Sacha's father was really unwilling to recognize his son's strength. The balance of strength between father and son had certainly altered. My own insecurities made me fear Sacha's judgment. Staring at this photograph I see my own father staring at me.

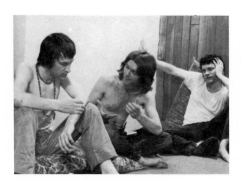

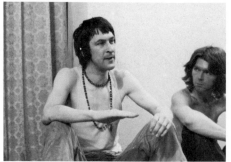

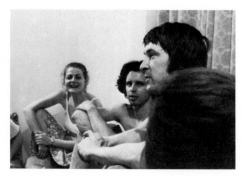

As though an end point had been reached, Sacha's interest turned from me to the rest of the group. During the next hour there was a period of play. For Sacha this might be interpreted as a time for free adolescence. Joining the other group members Sacha speculated on travel or a return to teacher training college. He entertained us with poetry, and finally at the close of the evening he organized an exhilarating group dance.

Our group interaction spotlights and illuminates our essential duality. I am inside, looking out at the world outside. The duality is a continual dialogue, a process of expansion towards the world and contraction from it, a joining and a separating and a joining again. Our aim and our task is to feel fully alive, grounded clearly in our own experience. We present ourselves to each other and in the here-and-now meeting try to trace back and work through the roots of our conflicts.

We are forever immersed in the ebb and flow of our own lives. Yet there is sometimes an intimation – heard between heartbeats and beyond the boundaries of the 'I' trying to grasp it – of limitless resources, always present, inside us and outside us at the same time. The intimation is elusive. Try as we may, we cannot hold on to it. We might, however, put ourselves in the way of it by taking a certain stance. I mean an attitude of innocence and curiosity, a love of ourselves even in conflict, and a willingness to stand in awe before the mystery.

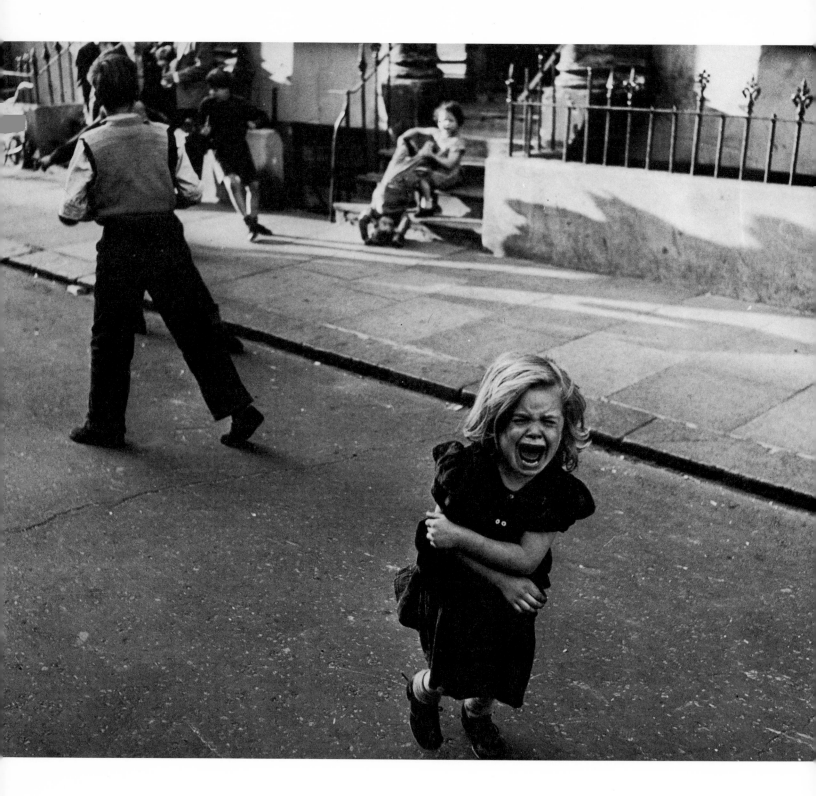

WENDY CAMPBELL

Wendy Campbell was staying in Los Angeles with her husband in 1970 when she read Dr Arthur Janov's first, and influential, book *The Primal Scream*. She immediately enrolled as a patient at the Primal Institute to undergo Primal Therapy. She later went on to train as a therapist, as did her son, daughter and daughter-in-law.

An experience in Primal Therapy

From time to time I visualise a second part of the method of treatment – provoking patient's feelings as well as their ideas, as if that were quite indispensable.

Sigmund Freud, in a letter to W. Fleiss, 1899

In the last decade Arthur Janov has developed a form of therapy based on 'provoking the patient's feelings'. The provoking of the patient's feelings is the essence of the matter, and it has become, in Janov's hands, a total psycho-physical experience. The patient learns to abandon himself utterly to the emotional re-experiencing of past traumata, both mentally and physically. Man has, for many reasons (some of them painful), found it convenient to consider mind and body as separate, but in Nature they are one. An effective psychotherapy must necessarily be grounded in this fact, for when a man comes to be deeply divided within himself, he is said to be 'sick' and can only be restored to health if he is re-united with himself and 'becomes himself again'.

Janov has also developed a highly detailed theoretical framework describing the nature and genesis of neurosis. Based on Freud's concept of repression and the dissociation of mind described by R. D. Laing in *The Divided Self*, Janov sees neurosis as a product of the pain which results from unfilled needs in infancy and childhood:

The development of neurosis begins when the needs of children go unmet. The child will be hurt when this happens and feel helpless to do anything about the hurt or the unmet needs. These hurts are often so great that the child must shut off their reality. He must repress both the unmet need and the pain of unfulfilment. This repression results in tension within the body which may be so great as to be reflected in psychosomatic symptoms.

The neurotic adult's life is founded in the pain of childhood. The tension remains in the body: the person feels miserable, and all his relationships with people are affected because he struggles to find in those relationships the fulfilment of his unmet childhood needs. The truth is that these needs can never be met once the appropriate time has passed, and the neurotic struggle can only be resolved when the pain is no longer repressed but felt.

Primal Therapy is the re-experiencing of psychological traumas. We lessen the defences which have arisen to hide the pain, and when the patient does not have to defend, the repression is lifted and he finds access to the unfelt pain, and therefore to the real needs which were unfulfilled. For the first time the person can feel the original hurt. This experience is usually associated with crying and sometimes with screaming. When these traumas are re-experienced, the powerful impulse for symbolic acting out and struggle is decreased. The person feels less tension in his body and feels better about himself. He is able to connect the early pain with the present-day struggles and his relationships will become more real, and his life ultimately more satisfying.

Anais Nin wrote: 'A great part of our life is an invention to avoid confrontation with our deepest self.' (*Diary*: Winter 1951–1952). When depression and chronic anxiety rise to the level of despair, what might be termed a basic overhaul carries the promise of relief.

Seven years ago Janov's first book, *The Primal Scream*, had just been published, and it made sense to me. Accordingly, I embarked on Primal Therapy in the hope of the relief such a confrontation might bring.

Primal Therapy begins with three weeks of intensive therapy. Patients are asked to be alone and to cut themselves off from all their customary distractions for these three weeks, during which they have a session every day with the particular therapist appointed to them; this session lasts as long as they choose. This period is one of serious and continuous attention to one's feelings and to one's entire life: a period in which one is learning the grammar of the therapy, so to speak, and possibly discarding some misconceptions about it at the same time. It is a period of looking within, for which most people have never had the time or the opportunity before, and it is the beginning of knowing one's self, of finding out what one's life has been about in the sense of what one has really been doing all one's life. The effort of the therapist is continually directed towards setting in motion a traffic between the patient and his feelings, rather than between the patient and the therapist. He does not encourage a transference; his function is to be both a bridge and a catalyst. He does not interpret, nor advise, nor console. For the therapist, the importance of this period lies in getting to know the patient.

Naïve imitators of Primal Therapy frequently fail to understand the underlying theory, and betray their incomprehension by their direction of the patient, and above all by the pressure they put on him if he cannot express the feelings that they believe he should express. Unending patience is essential. The patient must at all costs be allowed to go *at his own pace*, for when the therapist begins to force the patient (which is what happens when he tries to elicit a reaction he feels is due) the therapy fails – because the therapist is repeating the situation which brought about the patient's sickness in the first place: he is exerting pressure on the patient *not to be himself*.

In Primal Therapy, the patient is not encouraged to talk about his dreams nor to try to understand their meaning; instead he is encouraged to experience the feelings they embody. Abandoning himself to the feeling, he frequently finds that the meaning has become clear. In this way I understand many previously baffling dreams, and their implications for my life and behaviour. Sometimes a dream makes a particularly strong impact, and the feeling in it provides a concentrated clue to a great part of one's life. These dreams appear simple at first, but are packed with layers of meaning, and yield further insights when some new aspect of them is felt.

A dream of this kind heralded a nervous breakdown for me, and when I eventually understood the dream I was astonished by the strength of my resistance to understanding it, and not a little touched by the care my defences took to deliver a message in a tactful manner.

I dreamed I was defrosting a refrigerator which was exactly my height. I took some meat out of the freezing compartment and put it on top of the refrigerator. No matter how much I took out, there always seemed to be more. Finally I pulled out a bundle which fell open: it was a little girl who had been crushed flat, like a piece of leather, and then folded up. On her head was an Eskimo hood fringed with soft fur. I laid her across a chair, then I noticed that the frozen meat was swelling wildly as it defrosted, and streams of icy blood and water were welling out and splashing down everywhere. I struggled to deal with it, but it rapidly grew beyond me. I began to sob helplessly, but felt I had to manage it somehow. I groped inside the refrigerator for the controls and the knob came away in my hand. I cried out in desperation, then I saw the figure of a man in the doorway, against the light. I knew he was a friend, though I had never seen him before, and I cried, 'Thank God you've come, you can help me.'

I woke up, crying uncontrollably. A lifetime's frozen feelings were melting, overwhelming me. I had posited help in my dream and now set out to look for it. I found an analyst in London, and told him my dream, a dream as simple and obvious as daylight (though it was far from being so to me at the time). The dream contained the feeling, it *was* the feeling – a panic sense of being overwhelmed – but the analyst swept it aside and explained to me that I was deeply dissociated, etcetera etcetera. If only he had had the means of helping me to feel it, then he might well have shortened the years of confusion and wretchedness that followed. It was not until I was in Primal Therapy six years later and had relived many of the events that crushed me, that I began to understand that I was the flattened little girl.

Another dream which arose from my childhood had followed my first husband's death some years earlier. It was never repeated but was always there, at the back of my mind; a threatening image, wrapped in unease. The immediate cause was an argument with a cousin of whom I was afraid.

I dreamed there was an enormous Eye before me; it was about three feet high and from it there radiated a tremendous force. I despised this force and felt nothing would make me give in to it for I felt it was totally evil. I could feel my body shaking with my hatred and the vehemence of my contempt, but the force continued to stream ferociously out of the eye, and such was its power that to my horror I began at last to weaken before it. Very slowly my knees gave way and I sank to the ground

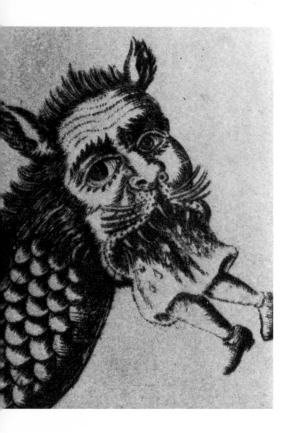

until I was feebly grovelling before it. I was broken by its force, defeated, reduced to the most abject and humiliating slavery.

I woke in such terror I did not at first dare to put my hand out to the light: the room was crowded with evil. I gabbled desperate prayers. After a while I gathered the courage to write it down as a means of distancing myself from it. I discovered in Primal Therapy that the Eye was my father; later, feeling it again, I had an insight that surprised and shocked me. It concerned a scene when I was four years old, of which this nightmare was the condensation. I had never forgotten this scene, but until I actually fell into the feelings the dream brought up, I only remembered it in a shallow detached way, as though it had happened to someone else (for the very good reason that the feeling was detached from the memory and buried deeply).

Although I had always become angry and helpless whenever my father and I discussed anything, I was completely unconscious that I had ever been terrified of him as a child. What had happened was that when I was four I had a nursemaid whom I loved dearly. One day she did something that enraged my father, and I remember standing and watching him as he shouted at her. I was beside myself, wanting to make him *stop*. I hated him so much for shouting at her I could hardly breathe, but at the same time I felt terrified of him and helplessly unable to halt that cyclone of bellowing fury. His eyes were huge and round and burning, they seemed to fill the sky. It hurt like a physical injury to look at them.

I have never felt such pure petrifying animal fear. (The first time I had this feeling, my therapist said, 'Look at his eyes!' I tried to, and instead hallucinated, for a moment, an enormous spider near the ceiling, and I heard coming out of me the short terrified barking screams of a small child, wild with terror. They hardly even seemed to come from me at first.) His voice rose higher and higher, and my rage and helplessness and terror roared together like a furnace in my chest. Then my whole body seemed to melt inside, my bones dissolved; it was as though hot lava spilled out of my chest, and ran down my body. I felt weak and broken. I ran to my mother and clung to her and screamed, 'I hate him! I hate him!' She said, 'You mustn't hate Daddy, you must feel sorry for him.' I had always understood of course that she was doing her best, but to me then, as I felt it, it seemed like the ultimate desolation. It was like falling off the edge of the world. My mother was my only refuge, and I loved her absolutely, and now in order to please her and be loved by her I had to not-feel what had just blown me asunder. For me to summon pity for my father at that moment was as far beyond my power as it was for me to get up and fly. Her well-meant injunction added despair to my helplessness.

Given any experience of this sort and of this intensity, it is truly extraordinary that feelings are so seldom recognized as having their own logical truth as being facts of the psyche. It is not possible to order them by an act of will, for feelings are not soluble in reason. There is nothing to do with a feeling but feel it: reason can only prevail when the swollen projections of unconscious feelings have been traced to their roots, felt, resolved, understood.

During therapy I experienced the terror of this Eye dream over and over again for several months. I would lie down in a session and my body would begin to convulse with terror. I would writhe and jerk in an access of fear beyond words, or I would scream unceasingly 'NO! NO!' with a feeling of desperate panic. It was as though there was a thick layer of fear I had to get through, and sometimes, to begin with, I hardly knew what I feared, though it always came back to my father, shouting.

Sometimes I only lay and trembled, my teeth chattering, moaning with fear, sometimes sobbing apprehensively. As a child I had always hated it if my father shouted or even raised his voice (and small wonder if it was the bell of helplessness that was being rung far inside me). This phase of experiencing acute terror was an astounding revelation to me. It was something I had never approached, even remotely, in five years of analysis, when I was engrossed with symbols and imagined I could *understand* my way out of the dark wood.

Similarly, I had been completely unaware that I had ever wanted to kill my father, and yet it had been a family joke that my response to almost any crisis was to murmur, 'Kill him, kill him.' I found out, with a vengeance, whom it was I had wanted to kill. The first time I realized it I could only whisper it to my therapist. He asked me to say it louder and it was nearly an hour before I could speak the words aloud. After a while he asked me how I would like to do it, and I said, 'Strangle him.' He gave me a cushion and said, 'Do it . . . ' and for three hours I strangled him. I shrieked my fury, my murderous rage. Sometimes as I did it I growled – I felt the muscles of my face contort with hatred like a snarling dog – and all the while I was in the very eye of the storm, the exact centre of the feeling. After weeks of feeling this hideous and exhausting rage, my head, which ached continually, began to hurt less and I fell through the cover of anger into the core of the pain. I began at last to feel how much I had needed my father to look after me, to listen to me. . . .

This total surrender to an early injury brought in its wake an extraordinary relief and calm, a feeling of well-being, of rightness, and continued to do so after every successful session. Before I entered Primal Therapy I had cried a good deal, shouted, expressed my anger, but I realized it had all been at a superficial level. It undoubtedly served to relieve tension, but having no guide, I had no idea that my tears and anger *proceeded from a derivative of the early trauma, and not from the trauma itself*. It is the origin of the expression of pain that determines the degree of relief and change it brings about. Where there is no subsequent insight into behaviour, no profound sense of ease and rightness, and above all no change, there has been no deep connection to the original site of injury. I realize also that the sense of calm and well-being arose from more than the relief of catharsis. It stemmed from a feeling of wholeness. For a while after each of those devastating sessions I was at one with myself; it was the first sign of the healing process, and the calm would continue until more of the old feelings were aroused by stress in the present.

The threat posed to a child by inadequate parents who do not fill the child's needs is very great. He is small and helpless and if his parents fail him he may not survive. If a parent behaves in such a way as to make him fear for his life, his most basic need – for protection – is not met. To preserve his equilibrium in the world, his defences must operate powerfully, and one of the ways they solve the child's dilemma is by separating the bad and frightening aspects of the parent from the good and caring side. I was quite aware of this from the point of view of psychological theory before I entered Primal Therapy, but as I found again and again, it is one thing to have a piece of information in your head, and quite another to find it out for yourself. The therapy was the means of making my own a good deal of what I knew.

It was not until some time later that I recognized how I had myself dealt with the dark side of my father by separating his good and bad aspects; and most vividly in the Evil Eye dream. It enabled me to love him and feel sorry for him, and to recognize and admire his goodness and generosity. The intolerable sense of my helplessness and impotence had spread like a stain through me, emerging as hot-tempered irritable intolerance. I spent my life continually acting-out, unconsciously, the fury he aroused in me. I was quite unable to see this until I had sunk down through the layers, first of rage, then of fear, to the need that underlay it. When I was able at last to beg him to love me and listen to me; when I crouched kneeling on the floor with my arms stretched up like a child, and beseeched him to look after me, not to shout, not to be ugly and angry, the child's words came naturally, spontaneously. Then I cried and cried as though my heart would break, as it had broken when I was small.

The Evil Eye dream also brought me a clearer understanding of how need operates all the machinery of defences in a child's mind. It was like going backstage and seeing how the stage machinery manufactures the illusion of a scene. When the parent is separated into two parts, the Bad Side becomes the Bogey, the Enemy, Them, and eventually becomes the fountain-head of prejudices which are beyond the reach of humanity and reason. The Good Side is seen through a veil of hope and need, and becomes the pattern for a series of projections that stretches from needing to see a parent as better than he is, to inflating the goodness of a friend; from idealizing a spouse to supporting the concept of a Loving God who will care absolutely for you. I saw why man has for so long posited a Good God and a Bad Devil, and the purpose that is served by a dualistic view of the world. Language is the vital means of defence, for it enables such separations to be symbolized more easily as names are given and concepts follow – and these symbols can provide the first steps into madness. It was interesting to note that as I approached the deepest layer of need in primals, my previous obsession with symbols withered away.

When I entered Primal Therapy, as I have said, I already knew much of what I found again, but the quality of the second discovery was so extravagantly different from the first that I believe there is no real knowing unless it is connected to consciousness by *feeling*. I had, to begin with, no conception whatever of the force and violence of the agony that lay concealed in me, or in other human beings. To feel, for example, in its purest form and for the first time as it erupts in a small child, the suffocating murderous jealousy of a two-year-old faced with a new baby sister is an experience light years away from talking perspicaciously about sibling rivalry or the Oedipus complex. Understanding with the head is a thin, cobwebby business compared with the ferocious impact of head and heart combined.

I learned more about myself in the first three weeks of Primal Therapy than I had in all the five years of solemn applications to my dreams and my misery in analysis. I saw that all religions and philosophies were man's attempt to accommodate himself to the pain of his existence, attempts to explain the unbearable in order to be better able to accept it. I felt the roof had been taken off the house of my life, and I saw something of how it had been laid out. In addition to this, my therapist listened to me in a way I had never been listened to before by anyone in my entire life. I felt that he heard me simply as a human being, without trying to assess me, or to sympathize, to improve me, or persuade me of anything. Nor did I feel he was trying to 'Do Therapy' on me. I simply felt I had been heard at last. It is impossible to exaggerate the importance of this, or of its effect on me. It was the first step towards enabling me to let go and feel what hurt me so much. Indeed, I hardly knew until then that what I felt was pain. I only knew that I was unreasonably wretched, and that death seemed inviting. My therapist gave me the kind of simple human attention that I had never had as a child, and getting it enabled me to move past the struggle for it. After a lifetime of trying hard in one way or another, I found I no longer had to try. Those first three weeks seemed to last three hundred years and yet I wanted them to continue. They were very painful and very exhausting, but together with the rising up of anguish, there were was always a counterpoint of relief. It took me nearly two years, at a necessarily far slower pace (after the initial three weeks), to assimilate much of what came up, again and again – and there was always more. In the first year it often seemed so endless and excruciating that if there had been any satisfactory way of escape I would have taken it, but I had tried tranquillizers, sleeping pills, analysis and psychotherapy of a more conventional sort, and now I had no other alternative. Above all, Primal Therapy made sense to me. Eventually, and gradually, I began to realize that the balance of my life had shifted. From feeling bad most of the time, I now felt better most of the time. I was no longer perpetually disturbed, tense, anxious, furious or miserable by turns, and I no longer searched obsessionally for answers, for I had found what I set out to get.

Primal Therapy is not for the psychological dilettante. It is an arduous business, and demands a certain amount of desperation if it is to succeed, for what but desperation could motivate a dive so deep? It does not provide a new heaven and a new earth, but it does provide access to as much of your truth as you can bear, or as you are ready to know. It provides a training in emotional honesty, and if you find yourself disturbed in the present you have in your own hands the means of dealing with it. It is always painful, and equally it is always uniquely rewarding.

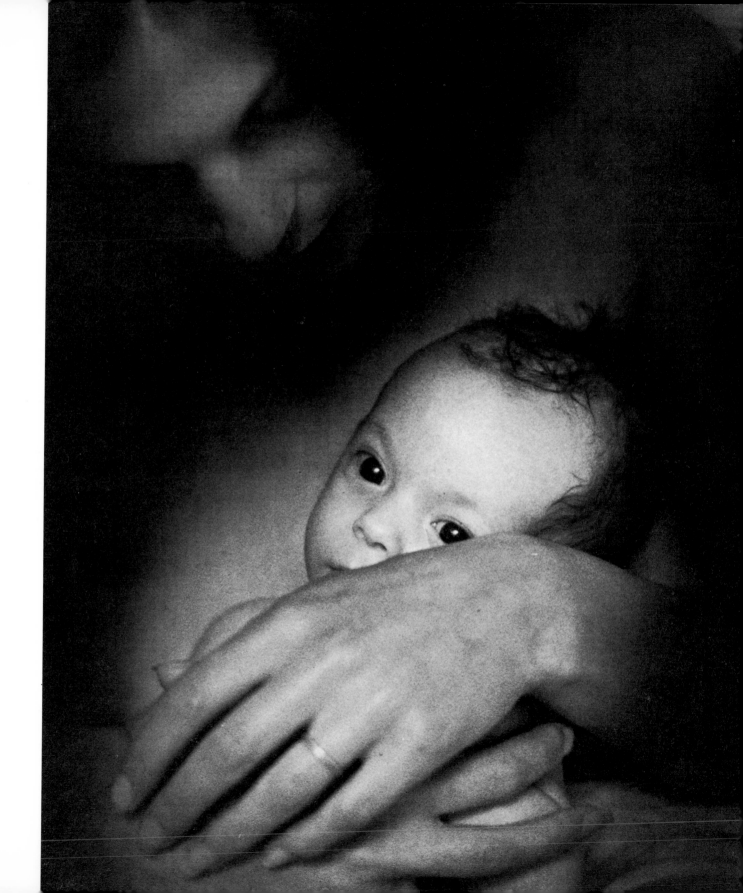

SHARON KRETZMER

Massage

There are many varieties and techniques of massage which range from the strictly medical to the intuitive and psychic. The approach to massage adopted by Sharon Kretzmer in this chapter is on the more psychic level: she wants to liberate the energy in a body so that it can flow more vigorously and harmoniously. Most of her work is conducted in Growth Centres, where she runs massage workshops.

My own great fascination with massage began several years ago in Lesotho, a small country in southern Africa. I had the good fortune to observe the last phase of the puberty ritual for boys, a ritual marking the transition from boyhood into manhood and one of the most important events in the life of the tribe.

During that ritual the boys were re-integrated into the society as men. It was a time for great celebration. For ten days, continuously, the sound of steady rhythmic drumbeats filled the air. On the last day of the ritual many of the villagers came up to the mission station where I was working as a trainee anthropologist, and we all joined in celebration. Local African beer was passed around in tin cans and the drummers continued to play. People began to move with wild abandon. Their dancing was earthy and sexual. Their stamping feet churned clouds of orange dust into the hot dry air. Suddenly an old woman was pushed into the centre of a pulsating group. The whole group began to ululate (a high-pitched tremulous scream), as the old woman gyrated faster and faster. I could see she was going into trance. Her withered face looked raptured and ecstatic, and her eyes were clear and steady as if she was in touch with something divine. She started to move around the group, from person to person. She massaged their faces and looked deeply into their eyes for several minutes. The drums continued and I could see that the others were going into a trance as well. Their faces were ecstatic; their eyes seemed far away, as if they had been touched by another reality altogether.

I was very moved by this experience. It spurred me on to explore the area of massage and altered states of consciousness. Many years later, when developing my understanding of massage, I became aware that a considerable quantity of energy can be transmitted through the hands and eyes. Certain high-energy states, such as trances, can be reached by one person and passed on to others if they are open and receptive.

The first stage in giving or receiving a massage involves simply slowing down: becoming more attuned to the natural rhythm, becoming fully *present*, totally in the here and now. The second stage is to become *centred* in our bellies. This is vital. Our centre, or *hara* as the Japanese call it, is the physical embodiment of the original life-

There is but one temple in the universe, says the devout Novalis, and that is the human body. Nothing is holier than that high form. We touch heaven when we lay our hands on the human body.
Thomas Carlyle

centre in man. When I asked a Japanese friend of mine what the word 'hara' meant he replied, patting his belly, 'mind'. *Hara* is the centre, the essence of our being in a spiritual sense and the centre of our bodies in the physical sense. It is located about an inch below the navel. When we are centred we are more aware and more sensitive. We achieve a state of stillness and total equilibrium within ourselves and within the world. More energy is available to us. In this state we are clear of thoughts and empty of judgments. We are without desire and expectation. Ego is absent, and we act as a channel through which the work passes. I do not do the work – it simply happens through me. Breathing, too, is very important. On the inhalation the person massaging becomes energized, his aura (the electromagnetic field radiating out from his body) expands and he absorbs cosmic energy into his centre. On the exhalation, this energy flows back up through the body and out through the arms and hands, thus maintaining a circular flow. This energy connects the belly, the centre of deep intuition, with the hands and with the *divine energy*.

At this point we are ready to start the massage. The secret of massage is that it is so simple to do. Everybody already knows how to do it. There is nothing to learn. All we have to do is to arrive at the state where we know and trust the wisdom in our hands and simply let them guide us. We step into the river and float, and the name of the river is love.

We approach the other person's body very slowly and respectfully. He feels our presence well before we actually start massaging. We let the hands rest on the body for a moment to enable trust to build up, to allow for the merging of energies to take place. The relationship between the two people working at this point involves a certain paradox. The basic state of the person massaging is one of receptivity and stillness although he or she is physically doing the work. On the other hand, the person being massaged, although he is lying still doing nothing, is in fact being active in that he has to concentrate – focus – and stay with the person massaging.

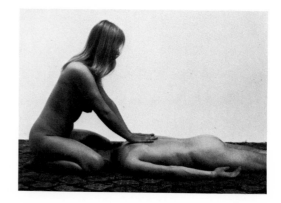

My hands
Open the curtains of your being
Clothe you in a further nudity
Uncover the bodies of your body
My hands
Invent another body for your body.
Octavio Paz

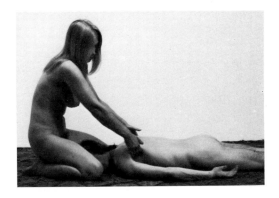 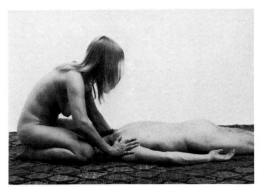

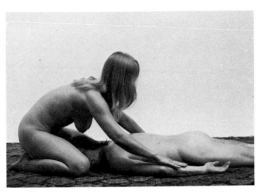 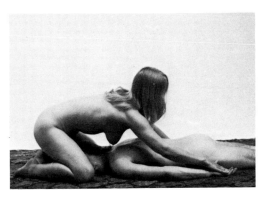

We start the massage with long connecting strokes, covering as much of the body as possible in flowing rhythmic movements. We move down the back and round the buttocks and up again. We do this several times. I call this part of the massage *listening with the hands*, because the hands are sensitive to the messages given off by the different parts of the body in the form of different temperatures and vibrations. In a healthy person energy flows evenly throughout the body and has a nourishing and harmonious quality. When energies are blocked, it is as if the natural flow of energy has been dammed up. The vibrations from different parts of the body are discordant and unbalanced. Some parts may be cold, lifeless, and have a dull vibration or none at all, whereas other parts may feel very hot and give a spiky and jangly vibration. For many people in the West, for example, where thinking is stressed above feeling and sexuality is repressed to some extent, the pelvic area and the genitals often feel cold and lifeless, and the energy around the head feels excessive and uncomfortable. In this situation we work to *drain off* the excess head energy and to stimulate the sexual/pelvic/genital energy in order to connect it up and to balance and re-establish the flow.

213

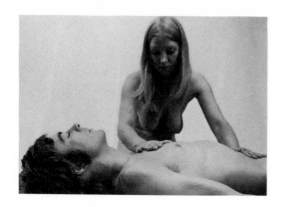

One of the ways we can stimulate this dormant energy is to massage deeply into the lifeless areas, massage right into the muscles and tissues. While we do this we breathe life into the parts we are working on. Another way of connecting is to channel energy with our hands, by placing one of them on an area that feels blocked and the other on an area that has life. Since one hand is a positive energy pole and the other hand is a negative energy pole a current of energy flows between the two hands and a link between these two areas is made.

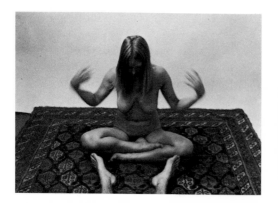 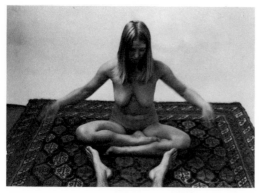

We tend to absorb the negative energy of the person we are working with. It is important that we be able to get rid of it and cleanse ourselves. One way is to allow the energy to pass right through us and into the ground. Another way is to shake out our hands vigorously.

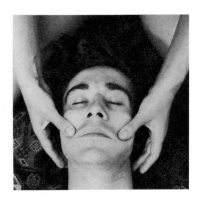
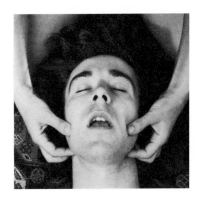

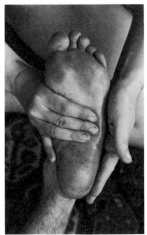

Contact is experienced on a very deep level, as though the whole body is being touched. Two people become one body, one breath and one flow of energy: it is as if the whole world and every living thing in it is one body. There is a feeling of ultimate perfection and bliss. In this state of trust and surrender we cleanse, purify and renew our beings.

In massage the legs and feet often have a special significance. The legs are our support, and our feet are in closest touch with the earth and the pull of gravity. Such expressions as 'stand on your own two feet' or 'hold your ground' express the value we place on being independent and being able to stand up for ourselves. When we massage the legs we imagine pulling the energy down from the pelvis and the hips, using long strokes, often having to work deeply into the muscles, helping to release tension. We pull the energy down to the feet and then out through the toes. We pay special attention to the feet. For centuries in Asia it has been believed that the feet are microcosms of the whole body, so that every organ and muscle area in the body is represented by a tiny area or point on the foot; massaging a particular part of the foot can have a beneficial effect on the corresponding organ. By massaging the whole foot, the whole body can be re-energized and restored.

'In sum, massage is an act of celebration, an act in which the experience of the giver is as important as the experience of the receiver. Approach it as such, and you will learn from within yourself everything else about it which you might ever want to know' – George Downing, *The Massage Book*.

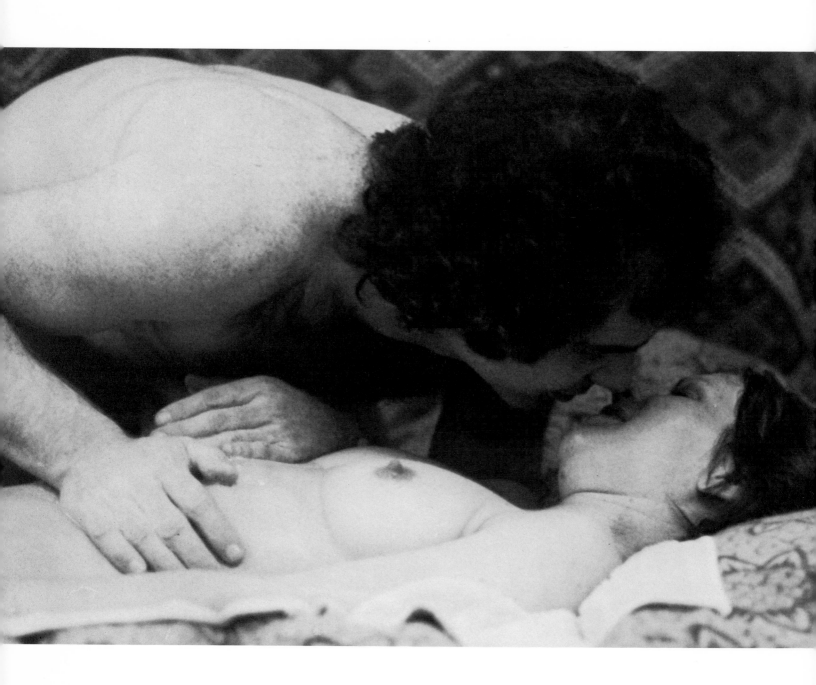

BERNARD GUNTHER

Bernard Gunther pioneered many of the massage, sensitivity and awareness workshops at the Esalen Institute in California, USA. He has written several books, including *Keep in Touch with Massage, What To Do When the Messiah Comes, Sense Relaxation,* and *How the West was One.*

Sensory awakening: Couples

Sensory awakening
is a method designed to
undercut the words
tension
habitual behaviour
goal orientation
to let you relax
non-verbally communicate
make sense
experience touch be
the open joy us
healthy harmony
you me we.

The following
are some meditation-like
experiences which
can help you to
allow recapture
uncover rediscover
the constant renewness
of each other.

The experiences here
centre around
feeling touch contact
sensuous delight in beauty
colour sound form
texture
rather than
sensual sexual indulgence
– this is not a put-down
of sexuality
one of nature's
most divine
sharing caring experiences
but only an attempt to
put into perspective
its narrowed distortion
in our culture.

Contact
of all kinds
on many different levels
releases
warmth energy tension
a more sensitive
human dimension.

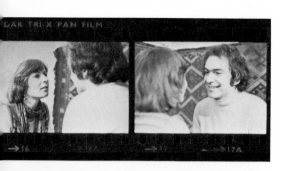

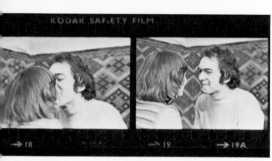

Your hands
are water
against my kelp body
warm waves waving
swaying foam forms
purple green blue
undulating
smooth soothing
light.

When doing
the following experiments
remember
love is care

Care for one another
carefully.

Generalized instructions
for experience/experiments:

all times are approximate
subject to feeling/circumstances;
don't talk unless
specifically instructed to;
to increase inner sensitivity/
decrease visual bias
keep your eyes closed
when asked to;
be sure to let your partner
know if he/she
is slap/touching
too hard or soft
too fast or slow;
after each experience
allow 30 seconds
to digest/experience
how you feel
before opening your eyes.

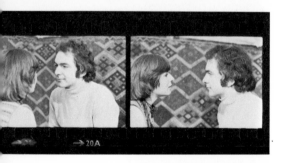

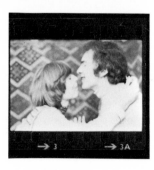

Being is now
when you allow
time slows down
and everything
becomes timeless.

Take your time.

Describe your partner
sit in a chair
or on the floor
knee to knee
and for three to five minutes
look at your partner
and describe
what you are seeing
start each sentence with
I see
do not elaborate
or have a conversation
stay with what
is actually there
before your eyes
then reverse roles
for the same amount of time.

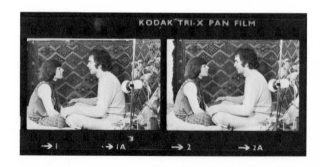

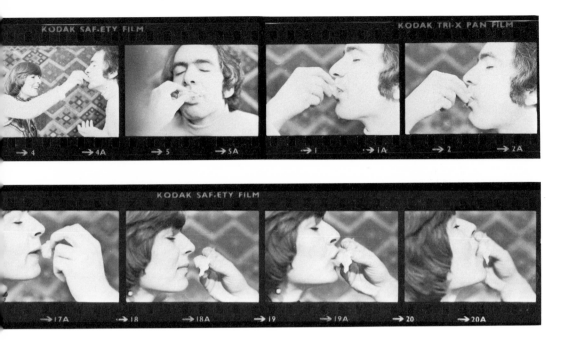

Feed your partner
one of you
sits with closed eyes
and is fed
a meal or some snacks
by the other
there is no talking
during the experience
now switch roles
don't discuss
your experience until
after both of you
have been fed.

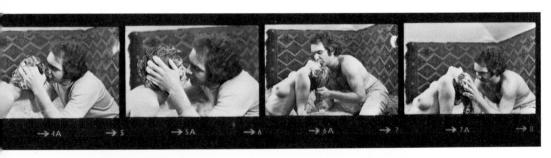

Give each other a shampoo
during the process
close your eyes and feel
play with the scalp suds
afterwards pour warm and
cool water over
his/her hair
towel dry and comb.

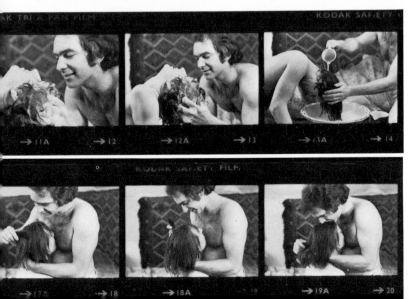

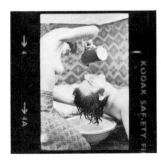

219

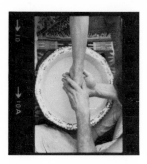

Wash your partner's feet
individually
first with warm water
and soap
then with lots
of table salt
dry off and
oil rub them well.

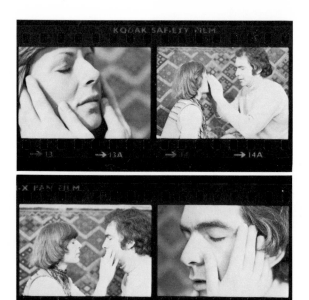

Sit next to your partner
both of you
close your eyes
and you explore
your partner's face
for three minutes
then open your eyes
and continue
your exploration
gently smooth touch
caressing away tension
afterwards take a good
look at your partner
and then close your eyes
and have your partner
contact experience
you.

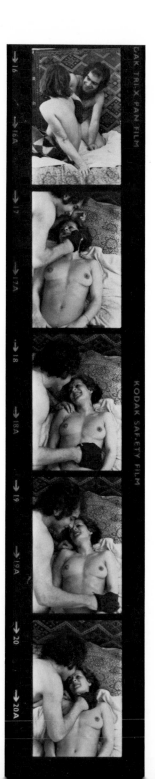

Your partner
lies down
and in silence you
wash him/her
from head to toe
with a wash cloth
from a bowl of warm water
take your time
after doing both sides
then change places.

Play master/servant
for one hour
for a full day
one partner's the servant
and in every way
accepts all commands
that his/her master
wants to convey.

Play the
'I see' game again
after you have
both had a turn
start a series of
sentences with
I want
tell your partner
directly what
you want from him/her
exchange roles.

Now start a series
of sentences with
I love
in simple statements
tell your partner
what you love
about him/her
have your partner do
the same for you
then discuss the
experience or
just be with
each other.

Being close without talking
and moving as little as possible
lie in each other's arms
for five to ten minutes
and feel what's happening
the warmth
the breath
the energy
between you

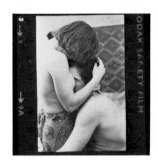

These are hints
reminders
experiences in awareness
of a sensual rather than
a sexual direction
that you can learn to allow
become a continuous part
reflection of your love life
together.

Soft silk
ecstasy
we are energy
flowing
in harmony
moving in
oblivion
and beyond
beyond
dark kissed night
purple bright
emanating
white star
bursting warm
tickling light
oh oh oceans
of love

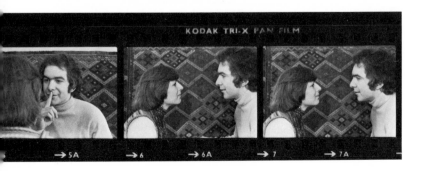

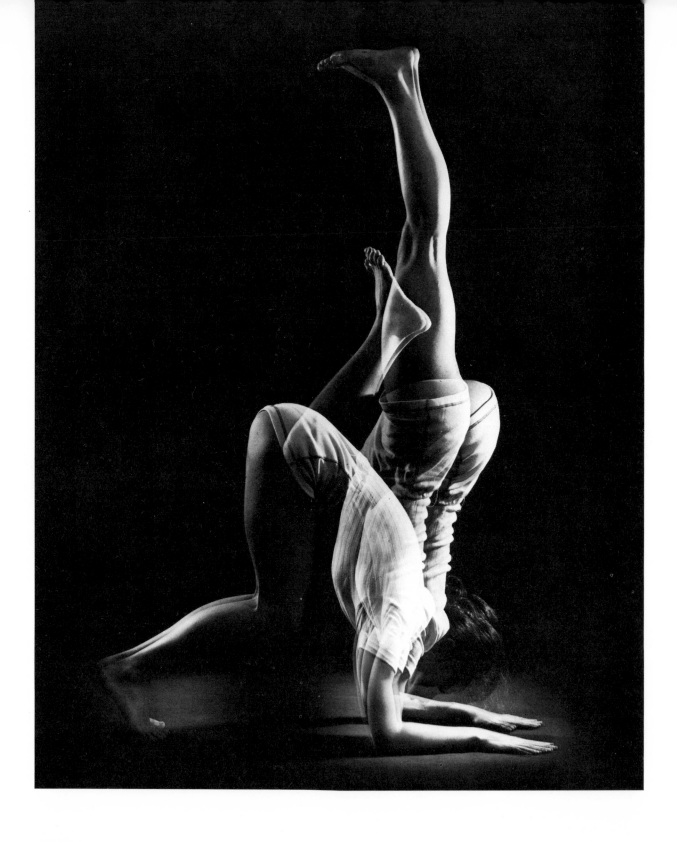

ARTHUR BALASKAS

Body awareness

Arthur Balaskas has successfully combined aspects of the Eastern philosophy of Hatha Yoga with a more Western approach to physical fitness and well-being that he acquired as a boxer in South Africa. His two books are *Bodylife* and *Newlife*. Here he emphasizes very practical ways of achieving a flexible and sensitive mind and body.

If we look into a standard book on physiology and search out the section on sense organs, we should find more or less the following: 'We are perceivers of the world and, fundamentally, our awareness of the world is limited by those forms of energy, physical or chemical, to which we have receptors to respond. Each sense organ is designed to react to one type of stimulation.'

Receptors are grouped into exteroceptors, interoceptors and proprioceptors. Exteroceptors are challenged by events outside ourselves. They include the sensations of sight, sound, smell, taste and the sensations of the skin. Interoceptors are stimulated by changes in the internal environment. They are vague but undeniable sensations, and include the feelings of hunger, thirst, nausea, fatigue, wanting to urinate and so on. These two types of sensation are obvious to everyone.

Now there is the third group, usually named proprioceptors, meaning 'self-feelers', which are stimulated by changes in the muscles, tendons, joints and inner ear. This group is too often ignored. The site of these sensations is the locomotor system of the body. The inner-ear organs respond to the movements and position of the head, while muscles, tendons and joints respond to stretch, tension and pressure. These all combine to give us the sense of equilibrium or balance and the awareness of weight, spatial magnitude, position and movement of our body in space. This inner muscular sense arises from the feeling of resistance opposed by any kind of obstacle to the movement of the body or any part of it. It is something quite different from the feeling of touch or pressure.

The eyes are often compared to a camera, and the ears to a microphone; in the same way, proprioception can be compared to a carpenter's spirit level. In your inner ears, muscles, tendons and joints is a complex network of tiny 'spirit levels' giving you your sense of extension, balance, weight, position and movement.

Proprioception is our most basic sense of connection to the earth, involving the body's relationship with gravity, space and the atmosphere. It is always there in the background. While you are reading this your eyes and thinking process are active in the foreground. Yet in the background your proprioceptive sense is active, making you aware of your body – of its breathing, for instance, and its spatial magnitude and position.

We tend to have a hierarchical attitude towards the senses, respecting some more than others. We value most those external senses that deal with people and the external world. Yet even loss of sight or hearing is not as devastating as loss of proprioception. Without it we would lose postural sense of our limbs and be unable to tell how they were placed without looking at them; in the dark we would lose our balance. Even though this sense may not often be totally lost it is often impaired by neglect.

We all know through sight, touch and thinking that we have a body, head, neck, trunk and so on, but how many of us feel the spatial magnitude or extension of our body inwardly and directly? Close your eyes for a few moments and try to sense your entire body, systematically; that is, turn your attention to every limb and part of your body. You will find that certain sections will respond easily, while others remain dull and beyond your range of awareness. It is easier to sense your hands and mouth or lips but much more difficult to sense the back of your head, or the base of your spine. The parts of our bodies that are used most are easier to be aware of, while the dull parts that play only an indirect role in our actions are probably not as familiar to us. For example, if you cannot bend your back backwards, you will not be as aware of those parts of your body which are involved as someone who can. In other words, to know one's body directly is to possess one's body, and to possess one's body means the ability to use it in action. The only time we possess and know our backbone proprioceptively is when we are able to move it fully.

Anatomists say that, from the evidence available, much of this proprioceptive information never rises to consciousness, which is partly explained by the scientific fact that overstimulation of any receptor can give rise to the sensation of pain and that most receptors show adaptation – if continually stimulated they send reduced numbers of impulses to the brain. Try raising your shoulders towards your ears and stay that way for a few minutes. After a while you begin to ache, so you stop. Now if, for some reason, you continued this for an hour, a day, a week, a month, until it was a formed habit, eventually you would have to live with this pain and the only way to live with a pain is to cut it off or escape from it through distraction. Your body would adapt but in that adaptation, your shoulder movements would become restricted and the sensations coming from muscles, tendons and joints around your shoulder region would be reduced until you felt nothing from them. It is the neglect of these sensations that allows us over the years to fall into bad body relationships and restricted movements – all of which cause stiffness, tension and pain.

There are many other positions one can experiment with, like caving in your chest, pushing your throat out or pushing your belly out, or tucking in your pelvis and so on. On the whole, we seem unaware of what we are doing when we habitually protrude our jaw, raise our shoulders, keep our chin up, bend our backs and many other less obvious habits. We are often poorly arranged in space yet we seem not to experience this lack of harmony. Some people are stuck in these positions and cannot get out of them. We have all seen people with crooked, bent bodies, shoulders rounded, hips tilted forwards, whose movements are slow and awkward, who give every appearance of physical discomfort and suffering. Yet they may feel little pain because they have restricted their movements in order not to induce it. A restricted body is, in fact, one that is in pain but without any sensation of it. Moreover, a restricted body is very vulnerable to injury and misuse. Sensation in it is minimal. It has no guide, no protection, and in a sudden bending or twisting or lifting movement muscles go into acute spasm and the body cannot move for the pain. Why should twisting, turning, bending be injurious to a body once well designed to take these functions in its stride? The obvious answer is that not enough time and attention have been given to promoting proprioception and keeping joints flexible.

Pick up a book and hold it in front of you to feel its weight. What do you feel when you say it is light or heavy? The weight or the pull and force of the earth's gravity on the book presses down on your hand. Muscles of your hand, arm and shoulder contract against the force exerted by the book. You feel the degree to which your arm and shoulder muscles are contracting. This sense of feeling your own muscles contracting against a resistance is again proprioception. Put the book down and the sensation disappears. Now go over to a table or, better still, a piano and lift it. Again feel what muscles are contracting. In that position, try to think of the day's past activities or try to become aware of all the objects in the room. It is difficult. Your mind and senses are hampered by the weight that your body is resisting. Put the piano down and immediately it becomes easier to think and sense. This exercise illustrates what a relief it would be if we could throw off all the burdens we are carrying in the form of restricted movement.

It appears that many of us are holding our bodies in a way that suggests we are holding up weights without there actually being any weight visible. A stiff neck, for instance, has very limited movements and looks as if it is holding a weight on the top of its head. The same can be said of raised shoulders. A bent back looks as if there were a force pulling it forwards. All body distortions or lack of harmony in a physique can be seen in the same light. It is as if our body were continually holding up weights or resisting forces through the action of contracting muscles.

How can we get out of these kinds of bodily situation? The answer is simply that of all our senses, proprioception is the one most under influence, through the fullest employment of our muscles in creating movement. But which movements?

Movements fall into three groups:

(1) involuntary, which includes your internal rhythms, such as blood circulation, action of the liver, and so on;
(2) voluntary, movements governed by your will, the most obvious being movements at the joints, which are actuated by your muscles;
(3) movements that are both involuntary and voluntary, like breathing and swallowing.

It is the voluntary movements that you can improve. They are within your influence and most accessible to change. There are two aspects of every voluntary action: the mechanical action of muscles, tendons, bones, joints, and so on, and

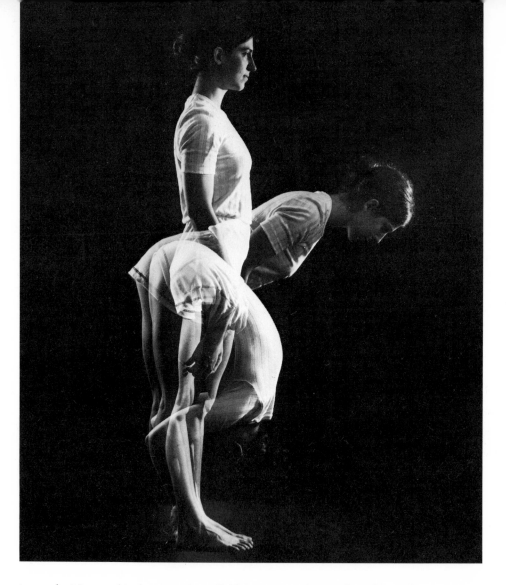

inner decision and judgment, the will. This continual interplay of muscle action and will is mostly unconscious. Every willed action or movement depends on the co-operation of muscle action, so the more efficient the action of muscles the more effective is the operation of will. But sometimes there appears to be a conflict between will and muscle action. You will a movement but your muscles do not let you carry it out. A muscle is then making you do its will, and so reducing the power of your will. Try a few simple tests and find out.

Bend down to touch your toes with your knees straight; perhaps you will find you cannot. Raise both arms above your head and may be you cannot reach the vertical without arching your back. Turn your head to the right as much as you can, to find you cannot turn the full 90 degrees, but only 75. Go into a squat position and find it very difficult to place your heels on the floor. Our joints are designed to make these

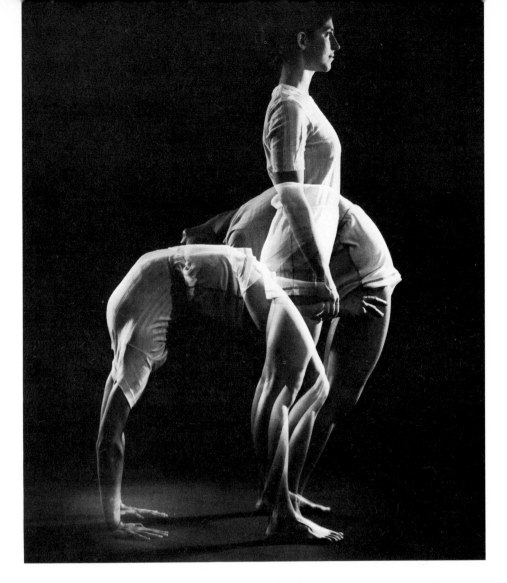

simple movements, yet we cannot always make them. We are prisoners of our own muscles. They override our will with a resistance or will of their own, which says, 'I won't.' This is then translated by you into 'I can't' and accepted as natural.

Because there is a perfect correspondence between the flexibility of the joints and the condition and sensation of the muscles acting on them, every limitation of flexibility produces a corresponding limitation of proprioception: increase the flexibility of your joints and you increase the sensations of proprioception.

Our joints determine our posture because they bear the weights of our body as well as being the source of movement. Creating movement at every joint will automatically improve the way we hold and support our bodies, bringing to them a feeling of lightness and grace. Though we cannot make ourselves taller or shorter, rounded shoulders, drooping belly and many other disordered positions can be

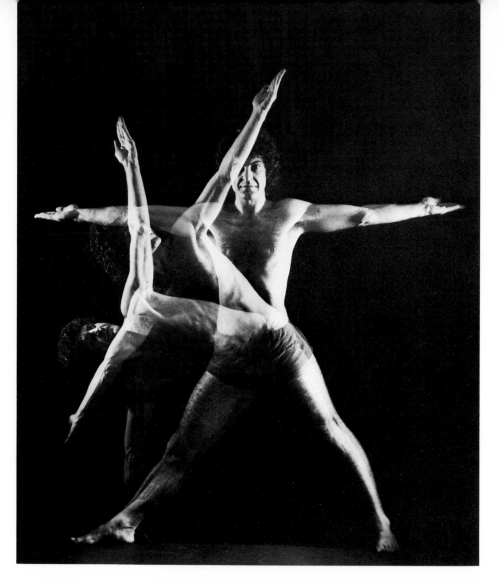

changed. The muscles which move a particular joint are changed in shape when that joint can make all the extreme movements it is designed to make. The shape of our legs and buttocks, for example, changes noticeably for the better when our hip, knee and ankle joints are flexible.

Our physical build and ability to move are probably more important in our evaluation of ourselves than anything else – much more than we care to admit. Difficulty in movement undermines and distorts self-confidence even if others do not notice it. Suppleness of joints inspires self-confidence by increasing the efficiency and aliveness of our bodies.

I suggest that we can help to make every joint in our bodies flexible and their appropriate muscle actions much more efficient; that nature has designed our joints to make certain natural movements and if our joints are unable to produce them

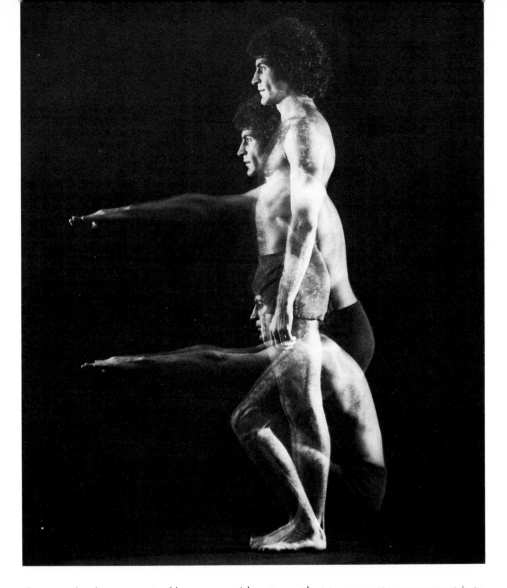

then our bodies are out of harmony with nature; that to promote movement is to promote sensation; that stiffness is deadness; that it is possible to improve our posture, appearance, flexibility and strength through simple movement techniques, many of which have been practised for centuries – for instance, in gymnastics and in the Hatha Yoga tradition. The techniques are quite harmless and not violent. When they become too much, stop. No training, specialization or equipment is needed. They cost nothing but time and attention.

There is no instant way of restoring a disordered body to its full potential. But if the movements illustrated in the photographs here are cultivated and mastered gradually, so that one stage can be carried out comfortably before passing on to the next, and if the movements are done regularly, there is no doubt of the ultimate benefit.

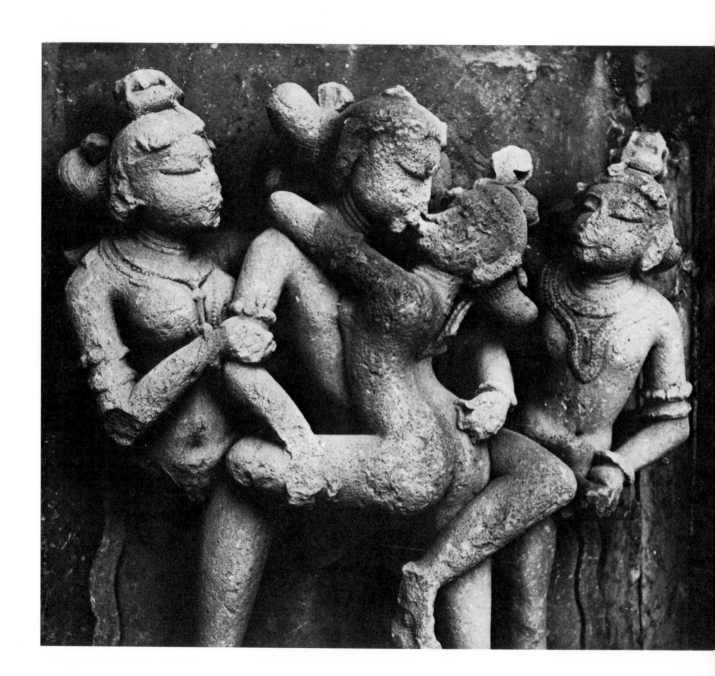

PHILIP RAWSON

Philip Rawson is the curator of the Gulbenkian Museum of Oriental Studies, University of Durham, and author of several books on Tantra and Taoism. He is also an artist, and a tutor at the Royal College of Art, London. In this chapter he emphasizes some of the differences between Western and Eastern concepts of self-fulfilment.

The senses of India and China

Broadly speaking, the Westerner takes it for granted that there 'is' an outside material world, which affects people through their senses, from the outside in, giving them sense-impressions. They then 'respond' to this outer world in different ways with different feelings, 'react' to it, and build up an idea of what the outside world is so that they can 'know' it. According to the way it has affected them, and the feeling it has given them, their idea of the outside world, and of the other people in it, will be coloured. One very common complaint nowadays in the West is that people are not allowed to use their senses naturally to explore the world so as to experience it fully and that therefore they are deprived of many kinds of possible self-fulfilment. The Indian view of the world and reality is almost exactly the opposite. So the Indian conception of the senses is also totally different; and the Indian view of self-fulfilment is likewise different.

What the Indian tradition assumes is that all we can ever know, feel or experience comes from inside us: in a radical way, each of us 'makes' his or her own world. Obviously this making is not under the control of our ordinary human will. If it were, everyone would make his own paradise, and no one would ever suffer. But people do suffer and suffering is an important part of the whole process; because the making of the world comes from a region far deeper than our ordinary everyday physical needs and desires. The point is that in India the senses are seen as a vital part of the apparatus for projecting each person's world outwards. They are never thought of as passive receptors transmitting external stimuli. Traditional Indian culture always looks into the person to find out how he or she (along with all other people) is being urged into projecting his image of an environment outside and around him. Control of the person and his projective faculties is the way to self-fulfilment.

But control here does not imply that nothing is to be felt, known or experienced. By control, in the Indian sense, all a person's feeling, experience and knowledge are concentrated and intensified. He can reach a point at which his appreciation of all forms is, so to speak, simultaneous. He doesn't have to wait until it's a fine warm day, or he is surrounded by affection, or can have a delicious meal, make love wonderfully and cuddle his beautiful children, before he can fulfil himself. Fulfilment can – even should – happen in the grimmest circumstances. And fulfilment leads to a special kind of knowledge which is not like the conceptual, discursive knowledge of Western academics.

Relief sculpture of the erotic joys of heaven, from the 'heaven bands' of an Indian temple, c. AD 1000.

231

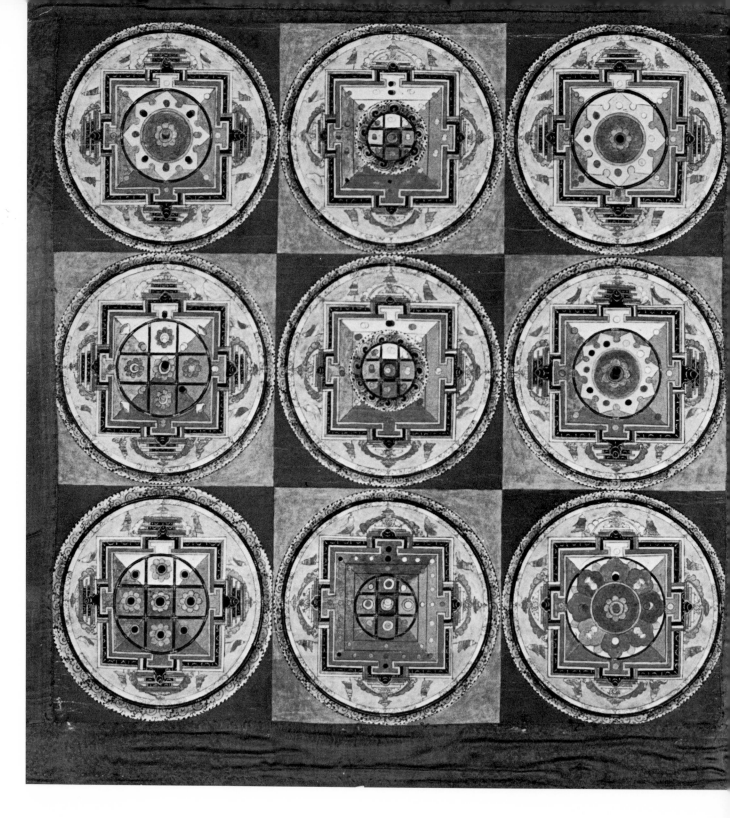

Everyone anyway, like it or not, is continually in the process of sensuous experience. Unless they are physically damaged in some way, or being subjected to 'sensory deprivation' their senses never stop working. The real problem is a question of attention and synthesis. Many of us are unable to realize that we are having sensuous experience even while it is going on. We aren't normally very much aware of the way our clothes caress us – unless they are uncomfortable. We aren't normally conscious, for example, of the whole world of touch; certainly we don't build it into a coherent whole, perhaps because our culture and language have banished this world from what they accept as worthwhile reality. So our conscious construct of our reality and the language we use to talk about it nowhere contain a framework of (to continue the example) tactile experience. What things feel like in our hands, what the difference is between sitting in the fork of a tree or in an easy chair, or the difference between one man's hand-quality and another's – these are real, and they should matter. But we don't have any words for them; and if we base serious action on such differences, say putting into practice our judgment of a man by his handshake, we may well feel we are being over-imaginative, even though we may well be right.

It helps if we realize that other people who speak different languages actually seem to know different realities, often because they have words for them and we don't. For example, the Eskimo have many words for different kinds of snow and snow conditions. To recognize them correctly may be a matter of life or death to an Eskimo. Some Africans, aware of their bodies in a way we are not, have names for different ways of moving, and even name the depressions visible between muscles. We do have the sensuous experiences; they are there in vast numbers in all our sense-fields; but our culture does not let us focus on them, or integrate them. The traditional Indian way to rediscover the wholeness of the person and his world is to look inward, to explore the depth and unity of all one's actual experience, to regenerate it into a kind of extended present moment, rather than to chase around outside searching for more and more sensuous events to respond to.

The meditating traditions know that by the time we are adult we already possess all we can possibly need. What we have to do is to clarify and redirect our consciousness. The arts can help greatly. But meditation is the final resource, with all its techniques of contemplation, concentration and integration. The seeming paradox about meditation is that its inward focusing increases the breadth and depth of one's experience. It does not diminish it, as it would if sensuous experience were just a matter of submitting one's senses to an outside world to receive as many varied stimuli as possible. The meditator, the yogi, the Tantrika, discover not just a higher reality, but the source of reality.

The different Indian philosophical branches share a common trunk, when it comes to describing the human organism and its senses. This trunk is itself the product of meditation, is always seen as the philosophical counterpart to yoga, and is called Sankhya. The Sankhya system is a description of the ladder of creation: the

Tanka with nine mandala yantras. Nepal, 19th century.

233

This diagram illustrates a version of the Sankhya system, developed by Tantra. The old Sankhya held that Matter, here shown as the work of Sakti, the female cosmic energy, is eternal, and Perusha, here shown as illusory divisions of a single male principle, is eternal and many. But the system, as here integrated into medieval philosophy, notably in Kashmir, sees both as generative functions of an original unity to which, by yoga or 'sadhana', one may ascend. This is done by reconstituting all the lower unities which genesis has progressively refracted, until the all-embracing and limitless unity of Brahman is reached. The Sakti–Siva pair in the rectangular frame correspond to Sankhya Mahat, the Great; the stages of 'self–other' to developing Ahamkara or selfhood. The gunas and instruments are the same in both older and later versions.

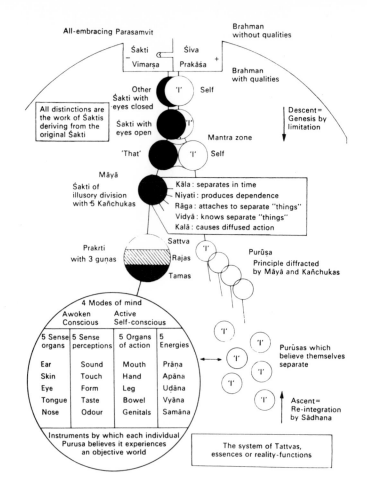

yogi seeks to climb it upwards, back to the source; the created world appears as the ladder is followed downwards. The yogi learns to follow it back up, to climb it to the point beyond creation. And the ladder incorporates the total organism, complete with mind and faculties, including the emotions and senses. Sankhya accepts two fundamental principles: Purusha, the individual self, soul or spiritual identity, and Prakriti, the material quality of manifestation.

Human experience of the world happens when Purusha becomes entangled with Prakriti. The entanglement blinds the Purusha to his own real nature and so he lives in a state of fundamental ignorance, believing he is a separate being inhabiting his own separate world. But if the Purusha becomes a yogi, he will overcome his ignorance and be able to disentangle himself, using traditional knowledge and appropriate action. He will escape the embrace of Prakriti by understanding the mechanism of her entanglement, and by disengaging Purusha from the grasp of each of her functions in turn, from the lowest upwards. Early Yoga did this by well-known techniques of radical restraint and one-pointed concentration. Later, during the early Middle Ages, Tantrik schools based on Sankhya actually worshipped Prakriti as the female function of Supreme Brahman; their rites and art set out to work on the organic system and reconstitute the original whole, in which both parts, male Purusha and female Prakriti, were essential.

All the lower functions of creation which limit the self to its passing material world can be absorbed into progressively higher unities. And these are not merely abstract, but true realities including everything lying 'below' them. The role of the senses in the full-fledged Tantrik evolution-devolution image is critical. Indian tradition explains the system in its evolutionary aspect like Genesis, from the top down; and this is the way we will follow here first of all. The consequences for life, art and yoga will be drawn later.

The whole of all possible wholes makes final sense of all the relationships which connect the world of experience at every level. It is the Ultimate Concrete Universal, the Brahman. It is the source of all existence; and to attain consciousness of it is the goal of all life. Being infinite, it can never be reduced, however much it may seem, in the human frame of reference, to be subdivided and subtracted from by Prakriti. It generates within itself the distinction between Purusha and Prakriti, between self and cosmos, so that each Purusha may witness something of the limitless landscape of possible reality implicit in the Brahman. In a sense, Purusha is the Brahman's own organ of self-consciousness; Prakriti is like a mirror reflecting back to that organ an image of the Brahman's own inner wealth. Thus the highest human goal of contemplation, mystical vision and union is what actually fulfils the purpose of the 'original' creation. It enables the Brahman to realize its own vision of itself: the enlightened human consciousness is, thus, the Brahman.

The ordinary human's daily experience of loving, suffering, hating, amounts to an active fragmentation of what is essentially one; and his personal libido is projected through his senses into broken bits and pieces of the whole scattered throughout space and time, attaching his mind to them.

The human senses are central agents in the continuous act of creation. Their 'elemental atoms' are 'real', but not what they seem. To look for 'Causality' among material facts thus has no proper meaning, only a pragmatic one.

One Tantrik version of Sankhya interprets the universal substance as vibration; its descending tattvas, or 'reality functions', produce overlapping patterns of ever more complex standing waves within fields of vibration. Hence the objects which we hear, touch, see, taste and smell are taken in this tradition as interpretations by the mind of patterns of vibration forming within the iridescent frequencies of Mahat, the 'Great' tattva, identified with Sakti, the Goddess as Power or Energy.

Yoga is the way of escape from the fragmentation of the tattvas, so that the human self can attain, first, the condition of original Purusha, primal radiant spirit,

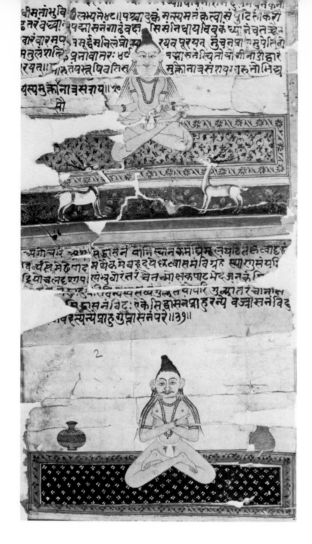

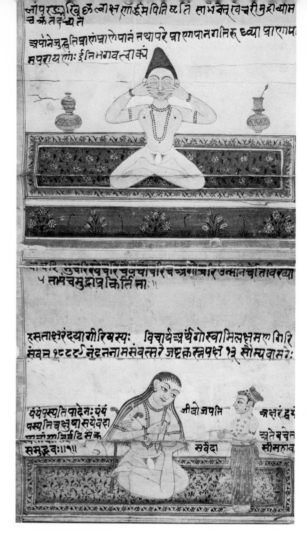

Two illustrations from an 18th-century Rajasthan MS. of yoga postures.

and finally, identity with Brahman. In its basic form Yoga requires that each tattva is 'restrained' in turn in reverse order. This means that the normal ongoing process of projection and creation is neutralized by the yogi controlling or 'pooling together' the energy of Prakriti-Mahat, so that it does not escape out through the tattvas into matter. A true one-pointed concentration of the whole psychophysical organism can reunite them all back into the whole from which they come, within the consciousness of the yogi. Then, the *Sankhyakarika* says, 'Just as a dancer who has put on her show [for her audience] ceases to perform, so Prakriti, having exhibited herself to Purusha, withdraws . . . hence the pure spirit, resting like a spectator, sees Prakriti as no longer productive. . . . "She has been seen by me," the former says, indifferent. The latter says, "I have been seen" . . . and no further creation arises.' The creation, the world and the body, are her dance, which absorbs the spectator's

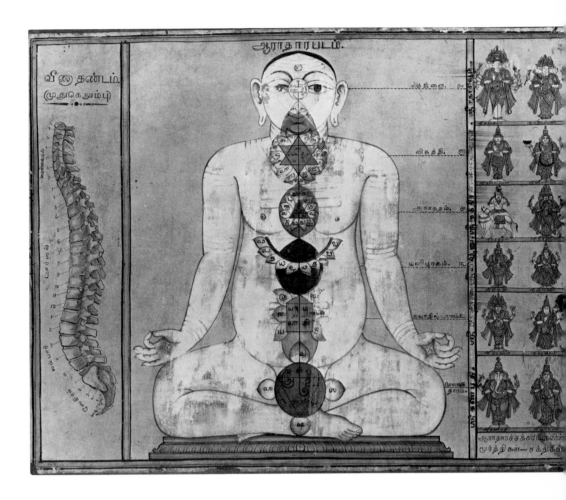

The chakras in the subtle body related to the spine and to the divinities.

mind, so that he cannot see what the dancer is. Once he sees her true nature, her dancing stops. This beautiful image has interesting connotations, not least of the generosity and love implicit in the dancer's performance.

There are important medieval traditions in India which do not understand yoga to be just a matter of 'restraining' or 'negating' the tattvas. Instead, they developed techniques for actually using the senses as an aid in returning to the primal condition of unity. These traditions can broadly be called Tantra. Hindu and Buddhist Tantra influenced each other.

Buddhism was a tradition which based its whole cultural effort and metaphysical insight upon four all-embracing propositions. The Buddha stated in his first sermon that all existence is suffering; suffering is caused by attachment to things; the way to release from suffering is by eliminating this attachment; and the route to such elimination is the Buddha's 'noble eight-fold path', incorporating right views, attitudes and acts. These propositions were projected by Buddhists within many different social systems, in various countries, which then supplied the environmental detail for the working-out of the individual Buddhist's release.

Buddhism had developed in India within a society many of whose educated members took the general Sankhya pattern for granted. When Buddhism migrated to China, and its texts were translated, at least one major Sankhya text was translated along with them, the *Sankhyakarika*, in the sixth century AD. For only a Sankhya text could make sense of at least one major development within Buddhism – its assimilation of the theory of the sense-fields and physical elements, the Tanmatras and Mahabhutas. In practice this Buddhist adaptation seems to have provided Chinese culture with its theoretical interpretation of the nature of the senses.

Buddhism, however, cultivated two other fundamental thoughts which modified the Hindu-Sankhya pattern. These were the psychological theory of the five Skandhas, each of which was given a schematic correspondence with one of the five Tanmatras and Mahabhutas, and the doctrine of emptiness. The Skandhas were psychological or phenomenological categories under which all experience presents itself: form, feeling, perception, intellectual movement, and habit trace from present and past existences. Buddhism taught that all phenomena can be resolved into compounds of these during meditation; and each of the Skandhas may then be contemplated as void, empty of any inner, self-existent character. This means that, in the last resort, nothing has any mark, substance or inner essence that distinguishes it from everything else. All such phenomena, because of their 'emptiness', are called modifications of the mind. For, like a rainbow, they only appear in a mind when certain conditions coincide.

This teaching both corresponds with and differs from the Sankhya point of view. It corresponds in general attitude, in that it sees the apparent creation of phenomena as being a matter of descending levels and progressive particularization; it differs in that it refuses – as the Buddha himself always did – to identify and name any transcendent principle behind phenomena, any theoretical unifying substance: Brahman, Purusha and Prakriti to Buddhism are mere empty names.

The kinds of yoga valid in Buddhism avoid any implication that higher 'realities' are any less 'empty' than lower. Sankhya objected of Buddhism that, according to its theories of emptiness and non-discrimination, when a Buddhist perceives a pot he should have no way of knowing that he is not himself the pot – as obviously in practice he has.

This relatively simple-minded objection has an undeniable force to which Buddhists have constantly had to accommodate themselves, by building an immense structure of negative logic. Different schools invented theories which attempted to explain the sense of separateness and individuality that everyone naturally feels so as to preserve the fundamental notion of voidness and 'mind-only'.

Opposite: a Srī Yantra, the most important of all Tantrik yantras. The outer triangles are occupied by divinities which represent the subdivided energy-self of the great goddess. Nepal, *c.*1700.

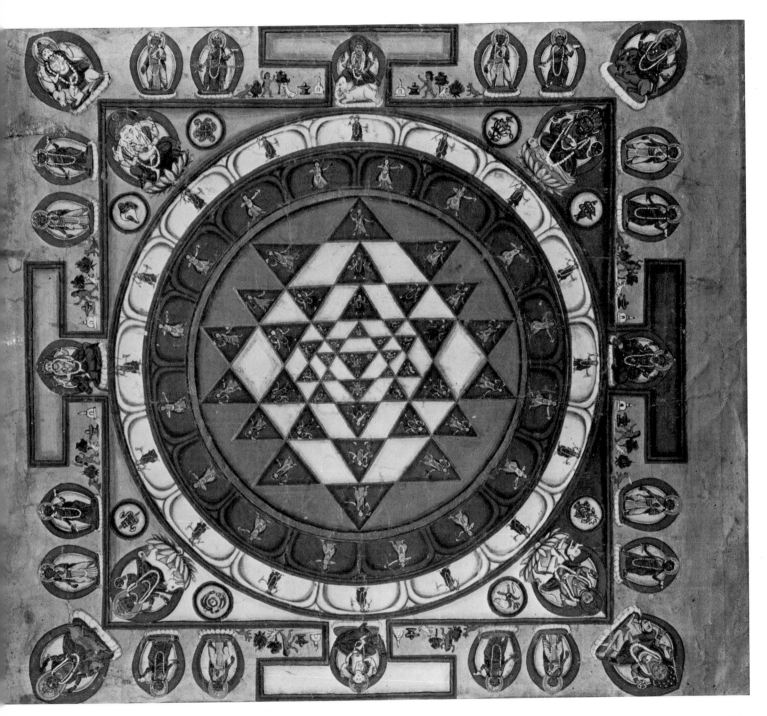

239

Zen is one of the best-known examples. But the most structurally magnificent of these theories adopted the Tanmatras (sense-fields) and Mahabhutas (physical elements) completely, and wove them into its system. This was the Vajrayana, a group of Tantrik forms of Buddhism, which flourished in north-eastern India, Tibet, China, Japan and Mongolia from at least the sixth century AD on; it vanished from India in the twelfth century, but persisted elsewhere into modern times.

All Tantra, Buddhist and Hindu, works by transforming the ordinary life-energies of the person. And so the popular image of the Tantrik master in India, China, Tibet, South-east Asia and Japan may represent him as constantly engaged in cultivating sensual enjoyment. He drinks wine, eats fine food, has sexual relations with beautiful women, wears silken clothes and jewels; he sits surrounded by paintings and delighted by continuous music in a perfumed, airy pavilion. To the uninitiated such an image was a source of terrible scandal, for it seemed to run counter to the morality of all the great ascetic religious traditions. But to the initiated it was a sophisticated allegory pointing to esoteric facts.

These facts were of meditative technique. To focus the energies which are normally fragmented and dispersed in everyday life across the Tanmatra-Mahabhuta-Skandha spectrum, Tantrik meditation requires that each energy be 'realized' to the full, before being inverted. There has to be something to invert. A fire needs fuel to burn. Someone of little or feeble sensuous experience is simply not qualified to be a Tantrika. Tantra demands that the Mahabhutas – the densest material phenomena – must first be realized at their highest possible power, imbued with the maximum possible feeling and energy. Then, when transformation and integration take place, the product will be truly potent. This is the meaning behind that allegory of indulgence. All the sense-fields and the mind's active organs of knowledge are to be first awakened and enhanced. Then the whole realm of actual experience within each sense-field is to be realized internally as a timeless subtle body, containing in condensed form all the compound 'objects' that once seemed to arise within it. This explains why Tantra took such an intense interest in all the arts, and in the theory of aesthetics, and why it recognized the arts as a legitimate means of release. For each of the arts awakens and enhances one or more of the sense-fields.

In the ear's sense-field of sound, for example, its Tanmatra, we all experience the atomic physical sounds of daily life, especially speech. But we are not usually accustomed to attending with any concentration to the dimensions, the depths and resonances of the whole world of sound. If, however, we do learn to be aware of all these, to 'enjoy' them to the maximum, hearing dry 'tock', 'spang' passages from 'whee' to 'doom' in their immense variety, attending to the overtones, harmonic colours between synchronous sounds, and the inflections or tunes of speech, we will be able to condense an ampler and brighter body of sound-experience. Music is the artistic mode whereby this sound-body may be awakened and unified within each one of us.

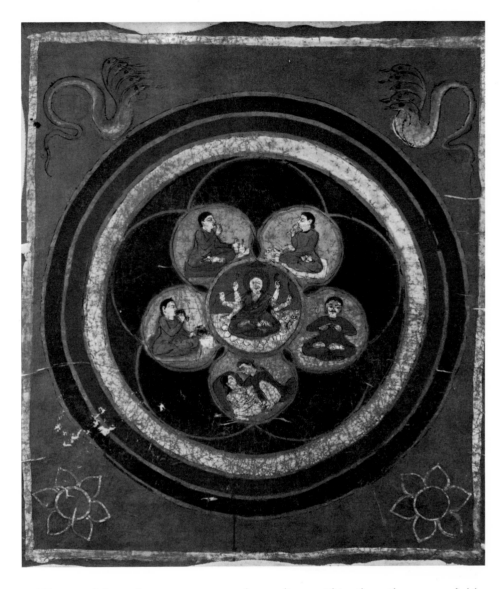

The five 'powerful enjoyments' (meat, alcohol, a grain, and sexual intercourse) round a figure of the Guru. Rajasthan, 19th century.

We can follow the same structural paradigm within the other sense-fields, especially that of sight, where visual art operates, but even within those of taste and smell, with their appropriate arts. All were highly developed in India (and in China). It is less easy for us to follow the paradigm with the sense-field of touch; for in the West this is one field we have more or less abdicated. We all must, as we have seen, *have* touch experiences: the Mahabhuta with its 'atoms' is there, but we are scarcely aware of it. Our touch-sense has been deprived of almost all perceptual reality and feeling in everyday life. We are not allowed to touch people – except our lovers, children and pets – or things in stores and museums. Tantra, however, should

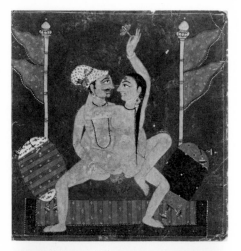

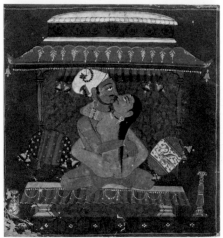

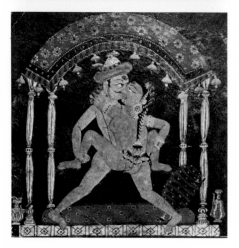

require us to develop this physical realization of the hand and skin, no less than the others; to vitalize and realize in ourselves through the organs of action all possible nuances and interpretations of touch: textures of substances and mobile surfaces, enveloping spaces, contained volumes, edges, clefts and hollows, enclosing and being enclosed. Indian Sanskrit poetry is full of similes and metaphors which awaken and co-ordinate the realm of touch. Indian sculpture is made as much for the hand as for the eye. Even today Indians use their hands as active organs of experience far more than we do. For our arts still offer us far too few chances to expand and co-ordinate our hands' experience of widely different conformations of clasp, finger-pattern, stroke and pressure.

It is in sexual intercourse that all the senses are perhaps most completely awakened and involved. And so sex is treated in Tantra as a fundamental rite. In addition, the physical union of male and female becomes a paradigm of the root-creative union of Purusha and Prakriti. But once again, the important point is that intercourse should never remain a mere end in itself. That would be to waste the divine energy, and reinforce the downward projection into the Mahabhutas. Sexual intercourse should be carried out, raised to a high point of delight, and its power should then be transformed, turned back up within the individual man and woman, to fuel the inner fire of meditation. Advanced yogis may not need the physical presence of an external partner; they develop within themselves a subtle body of the opposite sex which normally lies dormant. Intercourse becomes a metaphor for complete inner integration.

A lesser version of this whole system appears in the universal Hindu custom of daily offerings to a chosen deity, which was also adopted in Buddhism. The things offered each symbolize one of the sense-realms: bell for sound, cloth for touch, lamp for eye, food for taste, flower for smell. At the bottom of Tibetan Vajrayana icon-paintings, there is often depicted a derivative of the Hindu custom: a gruesome little heap of chopped-off ears, hands, eyes, tongue and nose, being offered to the main figure. It has the underlying purpose of returning all the realms of sense-experience to their source, by the route of offering and sacrifice.

The Indian theory of the senses was introduced into China along with Buddhism during the early centuries AD. In fact, very little purely Chinese pre-Buddhist thought seems to bear on the senses and the nature of sense-experience, in any systematic way. The early texts of Taoism, which crystallize such Chinese pre-Buddhist speculation as there was, seem to accept that outer things are in some way independent of man. This attitude, however, did not preclude later Taoism from taking the step back from this position, and adopting a scheme influenced by Buddhism.

The basic Taoist view of material reality was that all phenomena arise from interpenetrating and interweaving currents within the ocean of universal Tao. This is the true reality. These currents enter the organism through appropriate sensuous gates. That which appears each moment through the channels of the senses is simply a 'section' across part of the turbulent mass of threads of time and change; so at that moment the whole mass must be said to be in one sense non-existent. But the Tao is that whole, existing in another sense, intrinsically motionless but continuously vibrant with motion; changeless, but the source of all changes, which are wrought by the endless dialectic of dark feminine Yin and bright male Yang. The senses are, in some unquestioned way, gates open upon the changes, which allow a few of the Tao's currents to permeate the organism.

Man, however, is special. He unites in himself the polar opposites of heaven and earth. He has direct access, if he is not distracted by phenomena, to the higher world of being, the Universal Tao, which permeates him. He may become first harmonious, then one, with it. To do this, he must detach himself from the conflicting and turbulent sets of outer currents which are only details of appearance. This means that he must cease to experience 'things' but imbue himself with the 'principle of things'; hence he must become phenomenally 'non-existent'. The senses with their experience are held to be a dangerous source of distraction and confusion. Huai-nan Tzu, for example, writes that 'the five colours confuse the eye, making it lose its clarity; the five tones derange the ear, leading to loss of true perception. The five flavours disorganize the palate, causing it to injure the taste; likes and dislikes confuse the heart'. To engage oneself with sense-objects is thought to waste the body's vital energy (correlated with the sexual energy) and shorten one's life. And since the Chinese have always been obsessed with longevity, obviously to indulge in many sense experiences, as the wealthy and foolish do, is undesirable if one wishes to become one with the Tao. Indeed the senses are elsewhere called 'the despoilers'; and the wise Taoist is one who restrains his use of all the senses to the limits of possibility. Outwardly, he seems to eat little, to smell and hear little, to see no agitating phenomena; he wears rough clothes and eats coarse food. Yet he should not become addicted to asceticism for its own sake.

In the quotation from Huai-nan Tzu, however, there is a definite implication that, corresponding to each actual sense, there is an inner 'true' sense: the 'clarity' of the eye, the 'true perception' of the ear, the 'taste' which may be injured by the five flavours. They were sometimes explained by later writers in the Sankya-Buddhist terms described earlier. Indeed, the Vajrayana took root in China; and much Chinese Buddhist art sought to convey a kind of supernatural sensuality, an imagery of Paradise which symbolized the spiritual state of blissful enlightenment. But the original Taoist ideal is that the wise man during his time in the world, as himself a mere phenomenon borne on the currents of time and change, should not be distracted by all the other temporary phenomena that appear momentarily before him. He should sink himself into those true inner perceptions, which are of a piece with the Universal Tao, and tranquillize the lesser currents that run through him. The cold of snow or the heat of bodily water he will not feel; the desire for treasure and success or the fear of death will not touch him. All distracting emotions and fancies should disappear. He will then become immersed in the Great Purity which is the

Three Tantrik sexual postures. *Top to bottom:* Canchala Asana, Sukhapadma Asana and Yoni Asana.

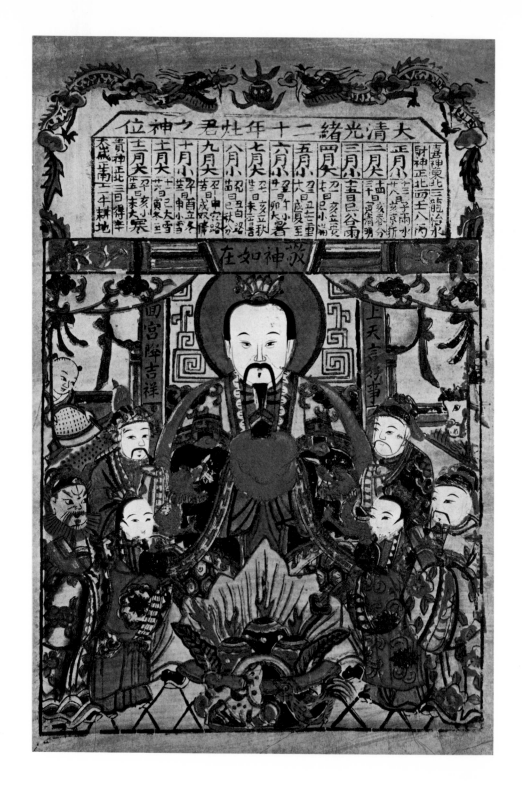

The Kitchen God, one of the pantheon of popular Taoism.

nature of continuous transformation, the formless essence behind all form. He comes to live on a plane of subtle sensibility, where distinctions between the senses and their objects cease to have any value. Closing his eyes on the world of sense, he lives in abstruse realms of the Tao, but seeing 'as though he were in a house full of light'.

Yet the Chinese have always devoted themselves to sensual arts. As well as music, painting, ceramics, calligraphy and poetry, they have long been renowned for their cuisine, for their remarkable interest in compounding incenses and perfumes, and for their sophisticated sexual techniques. There would seem to be a conflict here. Of course, at a certain level there is. For without doctrines and practices linking the sense-fields with the unity, like the Sankhya-Tantrik, sensuous indulgence naturally seemed ridiculous as well as spiritually destructive to anyone with spiritual aspirations. For two thousand years and more the Chinese ruling classes have refined indulgences and consumed luxuries on a scale so extravagant that the Westerner can barely appreciate it. They cultivated a corresponding finesse in stimulating the senses in an extraordinary variety of ways. There was, however, a theory of aesthetics which made it possible for all the arts – each of which is, of course, directed to one sense or another – to be treated seriously as vehicles for true intuitions of the Tao. This was partly connected with their use in daily and seasonal ceremonies, both private and state. For the purpose of such ceremonies was to harmonize the social group's relationships with the Tao.

An elaborate symbolism linked the forms and materials of art with phases of change, such as those represented by the trigrams of the *I Ching*, or with different constellations. But at the level of inspired individual execution, in poetry, music, painting, ceramics and sex, it was felt to be possible to organize and project symbolic forms which could convey an immediate intuition of the Tao as cosmic motion. Calligraphy is the paradigm. In the West it may be admitted that a person's handwriting illustrates his or her character and state of mind (not without objection; though objectors should open their minds more than they have to the Chinese and Japanese evidence). In China this fact is taken for granted, and an entire aesthetic system is founded on it. So when an artist is also a man of insight into the Tao, his calligraphy may project his inner state of mind into qualities of form which may have nothing to do with the topic of the writing. This 'meaning beyond the text' arises from an inner perception of material forms whose indescribable qualities appeal to non-sensuous responses – especially kinetic responses – in the spectator who has learned how to open himself to them. The formless essence behind sensuous form may thus be given implicit expression in forms directed through specific senses which do not gratify that sense itself. Hence a strange ambivalence imbues much of the best Chinese art.

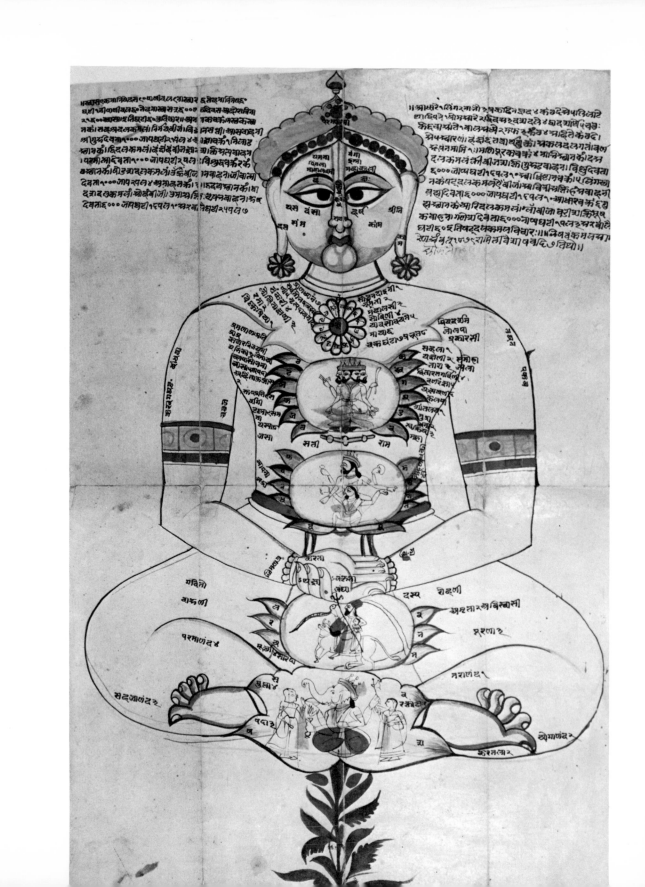

DAVID V. TANSLEY

David Tansley is a practitioner of various forms of 'unorthodox medicine'. He has written several books on the subject, including *Radionics and the Subtle Anatomy of Man*, and *The Subtle Body*.

The physical body is an energy structure. What you see is only a small piece of the energy structure and the whole energy structure contains a lot of subtle parts which you can't see. The physical body is just the densest part of it. I want you to know that all of the body is in the mind, but not all the mind is in the body. There is a large energy structure and the body is only the densest section of it, and every piece of the body, every cell, you can control, because it's all in the mind.
Swami Rama

The subtle body as a plant growing from the ground of the Beyond. Rajasthan, 18th century.

Extrasensory perception and healing

Consider the possibility that you may have the capacity to reach out with your mind to a distant friend or relative, and to see that person in your mind's eye as though he stood physically before you. It is a short step to then ask in your mind if that person has an illness, and if so where the imbalance exists within his being. If this experiment is carried out in a relaxed state and in respect to a real need, then changes will occur in the appearance of the individual who is visualized before you, and those changes will indicate the problem and the area in which it exists. This is one method of utilizing extrasensory perception, and many people are capable of doing such work but are unaware of their abilities simply because they have not taken time to try out such techniques.

If one studies the healing practices of past civilizations, especially those of ancient China, Tibet and India, it becomes evident that the physicians of those days employed supersensory faculties in order to observe man and the diseases that plagued his life. How else could the Chinese develop a system of healing like acupuncture, charting the twelve meridians of energy-flow through the human body, and locating with great accuracy the several hundred points at which this flow of life-force could be regulated and balanced in order to restore health to the physical form?

In those days, according to the ancient texts, men understood nature and patterned their lives upon the universal flow of Yin and Yang, keeping their bodies united with their souls in such a manner that they had the capacity to observe life with the inner sight we call clairvoyance. The sceptic, of course, may say that the charting of the acupuncture points and the meridian flows came strictly from physical experimentation and careful observation. When the complexity of this system of healing is studied thoroughly, however, it is hard to accept a purely physical explanation for the remarkably detailed outline of man as a series of intercommunicating energy systems that is the basis of acupuncture. As these energy flows in the human body were determined, methods by which they could be manipulated in order to restore health were devised. Needles, heat or massage were used at the acupuncture points to stimulate or sedate various parts of the physical organism, thus restoring balance and harmony to their life forces, balancing the Yin and Yang.

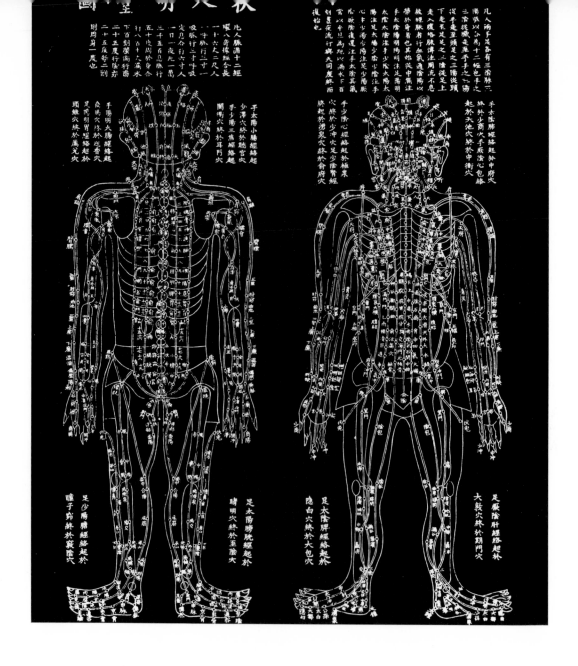

Medical practice in Tibet and India was also based on the concept that man was more than a fortuitous grouping of organ-systems, that he was in fact a whole series of interpenetrating energy fields which in more modern literature became known as the mental, emotional and etheric bodies; these, along with the physical form, were considered the vehicles of manifestation and experience for the soul and the spirit within. Each of these bodies was said to contain seven major centres of force through which energy flowed from the environment into the organism. These

Chinese acupuncture chart.

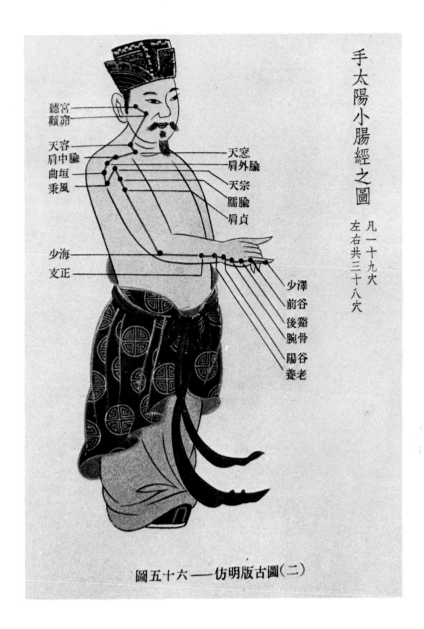

手太陽小腸經之圖

凡一十九穴
左右共三十八穴

聽宮
顴窌

天容
肩中腧
曲垣
秉風

天窗
肩外腧

天宗
臑腧
肩貞

少海
支正

少澤
前谷
後谿
腕骨
陽谷
養老

圖五十六——仿明版古圖（二）

Traditional drawing from China showing meridian and acupuncture points.

centres of force, or *chakras*, were located along the spine and in the head and were considered to have a direct bearing upon the health of the individual. Once again, these centres of force could only have been observed by non-physical means.

The ancient systems of medicine were inevitably coupled with the spiritual philosophy and practices of the day, and their disciplines of meditation and contemplation naturally engendered a high degree of sensitivity in the physician, leading to the unfolding of his supersensory faculties. This capacity can still be seen

249

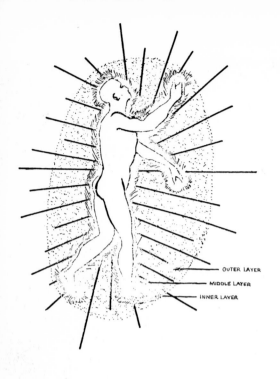

OUTER LAYER
MIDDLE LAYER
INNER LAYER

Transverse sections

Males   Females

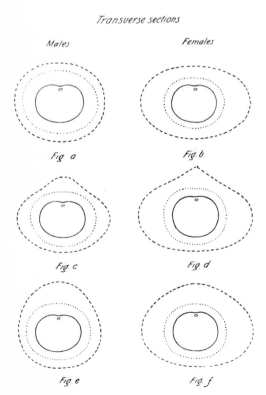

Fig a   *Fig b*

Fig c   *Fig d*

Fig e   *Fig f*

in the healing lamas of Tibet, who will take the pulse of a healthy individual who has travelled many miles out of the mountains on behalf of a sick relative. From that pulse the lama will diagnose with accuracy what is wrong with the distant relative and prescribe the appropriate treatment.

Despite the materialistic climate of modern medicine, use is being made of such inner faculties as clairvoyance and psychometry by a growing number of perceptive physicians, who either have these capabilities themselves or work with laymen who are able and willing to take part in such co-operative studies.

This field of investigation is of course not entirely new to the Western world. As far back as 1842 John Elliotson, Professor of Medicine at University College, London, presented a formal paper on psychic diagnosis; it was not well received. By 1866, Baron Carl von Reichenbach had published his findings on the experiments carried out with 'sensitives' who could see the emanations of energy from various objects and human beings. He did not refer to this field as the aura, the name now used, but as the 'Odic force'. In 1908 Dr W. J. Kilner, a man of excellent medical qualifications with responsibility for the electro-therapy department at St Thomas's Hospital in London, conceived the idea that it might be possible to see the human aura by means of a glass screen treated with dicyanin, a coal-tar dye. He had been inspired to do this by the writings of von Reichenbach and those of the Theosophist Leadbeater which dealt with the aura and etheric body.

Kilner's screens did in fact make visible an auric field around the human form, and after many careful experiments he published his work in a book called *The Human Atmosphere* in 1911.

Kilner claimed that the human aura had two components, an inner and an outer field, the inner one closely following the contours of the body and the other larger and more diffuse. In these fields changes could be observed through the screens which indicated states of health and disease. Kilner was convinced that they could be used for diagnostic purposes. Medical reviews of his work were scathing but in 1922 *The Scientific American* gave an enthusiastic, albeit cautious, report. Kilner was adamant that his work had no occult overtones and that the aura could be visualized because of the action on the eye of dicyanin, which made the observer temporarily short-sighted and therefore more capable of seeing radiations in the ultra-violet band.

Kilner's method provided a mechanical way of seeing the aura, but there are many people who can see these fields with no external aids. For the past twenty years Dr John Pierrakos, director of the Institute for Bioenergetic Analysis in New York, has been studying the energy fields of animals, plants, crystals and human beings by direct observation employing clairvoyance. His description of the human aura has a striking similarity to the findings of Kilner. Pierrakos says that when an individual stands against a very light or very dark background, and the light is soft and uniform, it is possible with the aid of a cobalt-blue coloured filter or the naked eye to observe a cloudlike, blue-grey enveloping field around the body. This

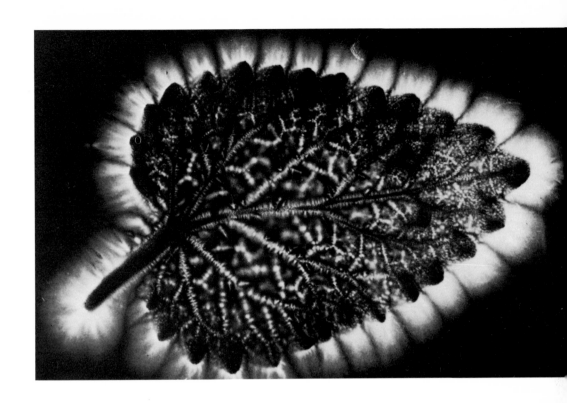

envelope is brilliant and illuminates the body, pulsing and expanding and contracting with rhythmic movements. It is roughly divided into three layers. The inner layer is dark-bluish in colour and about $\frac{1}{8}$ to $\frac{1}{5}$ of an inch wide; next there is a middle blue-grey layer measuring about three to four inches; the outer layer is sky-blue and extends a further six to eight inches, but these dimensions vary depending on the environment. In crowded conditions or stress situations the outer layer of the aura maintains this fairly narrow band around the physical form; in quiet, natural surroundings such as might be found at the beach, it can expand any distance up to a hundred feet. He goes on to describe streamers of white and yellow pulsing and flowing through these energy fields in a ray-like movement usually perpendicular to the body. Dr Pierrakos claims this energy field reflects the processes going on within the individual and that aberrations in it can express pathological changes. He has attempted himself to use these observations for diagnostic purposes in his own psychiatric practice.

Another highly reputable physician working in this field is Dr Shafica Karagulla, a neuropsychiatrist. She does not have the capacity to see clairvoyantly but works with several highly reliable sensitives who are consistent in their observations and have close control of their gift of inner sight. One of·these sensitives, Diane, has the capacity to see the physical organs of the body and can pick out and describe in her own way pathological changes that have taken place; her descriptions are clear enough to be easily translated into medical terms. She is also able to observe an energy body that underlies the physical form, and her description of this is identical to those of the etheric body in the esoteric literature of Alice Bailey. She sees it as a sparkling web of light in constant movement and says that any pathological changes appear in this field before they reach the physical. Perhaps most exciting of all is the fact that Diane can see the seven major vortices of energy along the spine and their direct relationship to the endocrine system. Her descriptions of these centres tallies exactly with the chakras of Tibetan and Indian teachings. Irregularities and disturbances in these vortices inevitably indicate pathological changes that have already taken place or will at some future date make their appearance in the physical form. It has been possible for her to predict the onset of disease by means of these observations.

Many who do not have the gift of clairvoyance have found that they have the ability to use the psychic sense of touch which is called psychometry. This sense may be employed by holding an object belonging to an individual and then interpreting the resultant flow of impressions that pass from it. Radionics is a method of diagnosis and healing at a distance which employs this gift of psychometry in a modified form. An instrument is used which contains a series of calibrated dials; these dials are set at numerical values representing the disease or organ of the patient that is to be investigated. A blood-spot or lock of hair from the patient is placed in the instrument, and the practitioner tunes his mind to the patient, who may be up to several thousand miles away. Through a series of questions, mentally posed, the practitioner is able to obtain an overall picture of the patient's health by observing the movement of a pendulum which is held over a metal detector-plate said to gather the energy patterns of the patient. In effect, the practitioner dowses for disease just as a diviner would dowse for water. From a broad physical approach by Dr Albert Abrams, who developed radionics in the early 1900s, this healing technique has evolved to embrace the concepts of man as a series of energy fields, diagnosing the condition of the chakras and subtle bodies and detecting pathological changes before they reach the physical form.

Treatment, like diagnosis, is carried out at a distance from the patient, giving credence to the concept that we are all linked in the vast energy field of the planet we live on and that this may be used for constructive purposes. Radionics, while most unorthodox, has its roots in medicine, and today there is a growing interest in this healing art from those who work in the field of parapsychology.

Just as the mind is used to scan a person at a distance in radionics, the hands can be used to scan the human energy fields for diagnostic as well as treatment purposes; this method is another form of psychometry. Dr Brugh Joy, a California physician, is one of the leading exponents in this field. Until fairly recently he was a strictly orthodox physician; then he underwent a profound spiritual experience which changed his whole approach to healing. Out of this change has grown his

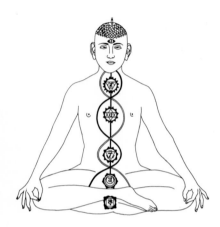

Diagram of the chakras or lotuses.

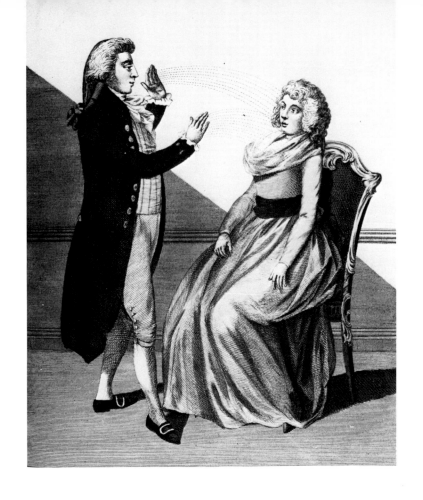

Projecting magnetism, or 'mesmerizing', from E.
Sibley, *A Key to Magic and the Occult Sciences,*
c.1800.

Four different ways of holding a divining rod.

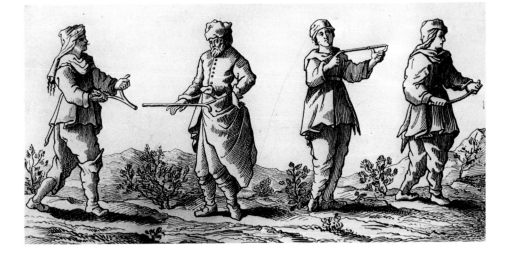

research into the use of the hands for scanning the aura. He began by scanning the liver of a patient, because he thought there would be a lot of energy given off in this area due to the great metabolic activity of this organ, and he found that he could in fact detect it. He then found a whole series of energy points tallying with the chakras, which at the time was an aspect of the human energy field he knew nothing about.

As he scans the patient's body a three-dimensional image rises in his mind, and he says: 'It looks nothing like the fields described by theosophical literature. It is more like cylinders of energy radiating off the surface of the body at both the energy points [chakra points or areas] and from diseased areas of the body. It feels like a bi-directional channel. They extend anywhere from a few inches to many feet from the body. I personally believe in the importance of scanning the entire body and balancing the energy pattern for each individual so that each point or area feels the same – an abnormal field is dissipated, or at least an attempt is made to eliminate it. I am now aware of twenty-eight distinct energy cylinders in the normal "well adjusted" individual. The seven chakra areas are only a small portion of the energy field.'

Of course, the hands can be used to scan a patient at a distance if the method is combined with the technique of mentally visualizing the patient. In order to illustrate this I may cite a case from my own experience. In 1964 the daughter of a friend was involved in a car accident; according to X-ray reports no bones were broken and contusions were not of a serious nature. However, despite all treatment and prolonged rest she was clearly not at all well, and I was asked if I would help. In order to do so I sat quietly, closed my eyes and slowed my breathing down; then I brought her name to mind and as I did so a figure appeared in my mind's eye with its back to me. I then mentally asked to see the area where the problem lay and visualized before me was a close-up view of the back of the skull with a hairline fracture in the left occipital region. X-rays had not shown such a fracture, so I assumed that the 'fracture' was in the etheric body rather than in the physical. I then brought my hands up in front of my body and proceeded to move them over the area of the occiput that I could see in my mind's eye . . . in effect I was moving my hands as though I was actually touching the patient's physical head, despite the fact that she was over twenty miles away at the time. As I worked in this way the 'fracture' began to fade out just as though it were a chalk line being erased from a blackboard. Within a week the patient had totally recovered and returned to her studies.

I am not clairvoyant, and I do not see auras, but I firmly believe that the method described here does bring the practitioner into contact with his patient at another level of reality that lies beyond the physical; that at that level the intention to heal brings about a flow of energies that can be mentally directed to do whatever the practitioner wants them to do; and that by this method he can in a very creative way affect matter. Visualization is of course the key to such work, bearing in mind the ancient axiom that energy follows thought. The sceptic will naturally say it's all imagination, it's all in the mind. To this I would reply that the imagination is an incredibly powerful means of manipulating and directing energy and that the mind is as yet an untapped source of potential in the field of healing.

In 1974 the American healer Dr Olga Worrall carried out experiments to see if the energy employed in this form of healing could be detected in a scientific manner. A Wilson cloud chamber, which is normally used to make visible the pathways of high-energy nuclear particles, was set up in the physics department of Agnes Scott College, Atlanta, Georgia. Olga Worrall placed her hands at each end of the apparatus without touching it, then visualized the healing energies flowing from her hands into the chamber. Within 30 seconds the mist began to pulsate and dark waves became visible. A shift in the position of her hands altered the flow of energy through the chamber accordingly. Soon afterwards, the experiment was repeated, but this time Dr Worrall and the chamber were 600 miles apart. By simply visualizing her hands at each end of the chamber and mentally directing energy through it, the same results were obtained. Here was scientifically measurable proof that potentially healing energy directed by the mind of the healer did in fact have an effect at a distance.

Clearly, despite or perhaps because of the increasingly materialistic and mechanistic approach to health by medicine, there is a pattern emerging which suggests that the methods of diagnosis and concepts of healing as employed by physicians of past civilizations are coming to the attention of individuals in the healing arts today. Perhaps we shall see an ever-increasing number of sensitives entering as qualified practitioners into the ranks of the healing professions, who will demonstrate through the use of their inner senses the reality of extrasensory perception and its role in medicine.

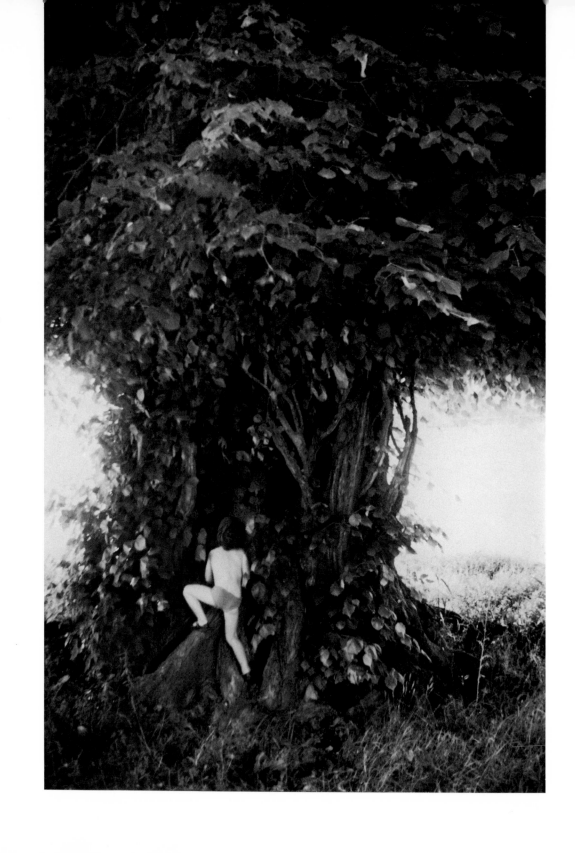

LYALL WATSON

Author of *Supernature, The Romeo Error,* and *Gifts of Unknown Things,* Lyall Watson is a naturalist who is no longer interested in the established explanations. In this chapter he urges us to look into ourselves and rediscover a knowledge, an awareness, a potential, a sensitivity that we do not normally allow ourselves to recognize.

I see all, am all, all.
I leap along the line of the horizon hill,
I am a cloud in the high sky,
I trace the veins of intricate fern.
In the dark ivy wall the wren's world
Soft to bird breast nest of round eggs is mine,
Mine in the rowan-tree the blackbird's thought
Inviolate in leaves ensphered.
I am bird-world, leaf-life, I am wasp-world hung
Under low berry-branch of hidden thorn,
Friable paper-world humming with hate,
Moss-thought, rain-thought, stone still thought on
*   the hill*
Never, never, never will I go home to be a child.
    Kathleen Rain

Many realities

How does it really feel?

You and I both know, because we have felt it. But telling about this feeling is not so easy. Something happens to an experience in translation that distorts it beyond all recognition. Our grammar and goals are incompatible with certain kinds of truth. There are levels of personal experience far too mysterious for totally objective common sense. There are things that cannot be known by exercise only of the scientific method that has stood us in such good stead in other areas.

This is not a new problem. Ever since we first began to think about ourselves in relation to our surroundings, we have been faced with the difficulty of reconciling natural knowing, the way people feel, with the current concepts embodied in formal education. And all too often the puzzle has been resolved in the same restrictive way – by compromise, by reaching an agreement.

Many of these mutual understandings have proved to be valuable and durable. Without them it would have been impossible to formulate any rules or laws, and we would have made no legal or technological progress whatsoever. But we have been playing the game for so long now we tend to forget that the first moves were purely arbitrary, that the entire structure rests on nothing more solid than an agreement – a convention, an artificial standard which bears no more relation to the true nature of reality than the limited wavelengths of visible light do to the entire electromagnetic spectrum.

The simile is an exact one. Our panoply of senses have become subordinated by one of their number, by the system that has been specifically designed to detect radiations whose wavelength is restricted to the small area around half a micron. The eye is an extraordinary organ. It not only isolates these particular signals from the mass of environmental information, but goes on to make further restrictive selections based purely on a program that determines what we think we ought to see. The eye is part of the brain and under their joint dictatorship, all information is translated into a visual code. Inner experiences are expected to conform to outer perceptions. They are supposed to stick to the agreement. If they fail to correspond, then we dismiss them as hallucinations. Anything that cannot be clearly seen, has not been sensed, it is nonsense.

Science insists on seeing how things work, it demands 'observations' – visual experiences encoded in verbal reports. It ignores sensations that avoid easy visual description. Anything that evades verbal classification falls outside the scope of the agreement, is labelled impossible and discarded. Whole areas of experience are left virtually unexplored just because they conflict with current orthodoxy. It begins to look more and more as though we have been deliberately deluding ourselves. And that is absurd. Our scientific theories have served us well. Many have stood the test of experience for long periods of time, while others, that have been found to be wanting, have been superseded. But the time has come now to discard many more – not because we have decided to make other experiments, but because we have made up our minds to have different experiences.

One area of science, that concerned with particle physics, has already run headlong into the dilemma with the discovery of a measurement problem at subatomic levels. It has proved to be impossible to determine exactly the position and momentum of any body at a single instant in time. No matter how hard we try, there are some things that we can never know. Not because we are inept, but simply because we are involved. By being there, by taking a measurement or making an observation, we change the situation.

In the words of quantum mechanics, an observer collapses the system under scrutiny into one of its infinite number of component states. Without the observer, there is no description – and with the observer, there can be no such thing as an objective experiment. Whether we like it or not, we are intimately involved in all reality, and its revealed nature depends to a very great extent on our agreements about it. We make reality with our minds. And, if this is true, then we can also break it with our minds. We can change the way things are by changing our minds about them.

Children do it very easily. In the first few years of life, there are no fixed agreements. Everything has a magical quality. Before minds ossify into the channels prescribed by the current formula, all events are shrouded in mystery. They take place in a world where anything is possible. Objects appear and disappear, the sun rises and sets, people come and go. As a child's mind moves to take all these things into account, it begins to make connections and to draw inferences without having access to all the facts. This leads to conclusions which to us seem bizarre and totally delusional. Holding your breath for a long time is a good way to make the sun stay behind a cloud. Counting very quickly up to twenty while you stand on one leg with your eyes closed is how to make a wish come true. Thinking about a burst tyre is enough to cause it actually to happen – isn't it?

Can you really be certain that there is no causal connection? Do you know beyond doubt that your thoughts have no influence over your environment? No modern physicist shares your certitude. The most advanced cosmologies all include consciousness as an active participating factor. And the new equations are very much like the old beliefs of children everywhere. Undogmatic young minds are

The great extension of our experience in recent years has brought to light the insufficiency of our simple mechanical conceptions and, as a consequence, has shaken the foundation on which the customary interpretation of observation was based.
Niels Bohr

much concerned with magic, and as a result they arrive at descriptions of reality which to us seem faulty, but in the final analysis prove to be far more meaningful than those we contrive by the elaborate exercise of logic and contingent mathematics. It seems that merely by admitting the possibility of unlikely events, you increase the probability of their occurrence. And the cosmos is filled with unlikely things.

In Toronto, a group of people started an experiment in which they attempted to experience a collective hallucination. They tried to conjure up a ghost. Not a spectre of a long-dead individual, but the vision of a completely fictitious seventeenth-century nobleman. They called him Philip and compiled a detailed imaginary biography for him beforehand so that his manifestation, if it should take place, could not be confused with that of a real spirit. For two years they struggled, but nothing happened until a session when several members of the group were involved in some child-like horseplay.

Then the table round which they were seated began to rock.

They have still not seen Philip, but today, by consciously attempting to behave like children, by singing silly songs and regressing to the point where their communal thinking once again takes on magical qualities, they can produce psychokinetic phenomena at will. While I sat with the Philip group one evening, they became involved in a long and splendidly bawdy conversation with their imaginary ghost, which ended only when a very heavy table rose until all its four legs were off the ground and pursued the photographer from an American magazine round the room until it had him pinned to the wall.

No single person in that group has conscious control over what will happen and not one of them is indispensable. All they need is a quorum. It is psychokinesis by committee, and by communal agreement that such things are possible. The conscious acceptance of such an agreement is simplified by the invention of the projection they call Philip, and facilitated by suspension of normal everyday rules and adult responsibilities in their deliberately childlike approach. But what they have shown is that any group of people, ordinary folk without a single psychic pretension between them, can produce, on demand and at will, well-developed paranormal phenomena.

Anyone can get round the rules of traditional science, anyone can break the terms of the agreement, simply by pretending that they don't exist.

I believe it is important that we should do this. There is more at stake than children's games. The things I am looking for are impossible to see. I feel that insight in this situation is more important than sight, and what my instinct tells me is that we need the strange ones, the special people, the ones who keep on breaking the rules. We need the child prodigies who begin composing music at the age of four, the 'idiot savants' who cannot read or write but can work out square roots to the fifth decimal place in seconds, the metal-benders and the ones who see things.

Instead of getting stuck on surface detail, they respond in some way to the

"Osses,' said the coachman to Tom Brown, "as to wear blinkers, so's they only see wot's in front of 'em: and that's the safest plan 'umble folk like you and me.' Nature seems to have worked on much the same principle. Our sense organs and our brains operate as an intricate kind of filter which limits and directs the mind's clairvoyant powers, so that under normal conditions attention is concentrated on just those objects or situations that are of biological importance for the survival of the organism and its species.
Sir Cyril Burt

259

underlying form of things. They are closer to the roots of being, more touched by continuity. They practise sensory blending, they dance to the light and find inspiration in the earth. We are all a little like that, we all have access to power, but I think we need their example to make it work. We need to know them better.

At King's College in London, Professor John Taylor has been making heroic efforts to get the framework of classical physics to bend far enough to accommodate unexpected phenomena. He began working with Uri Geller and went on to perform an elegant series of experiments with children who, having seen the Israeli psychic perform on television, started to repeat his mental metal-bending feats for themselves. In the past few years this group have quite independently come up with a number of variations of their own invention, and Taylor has followed them every step of the way, recording and analysing, setting up experiments to eliminate the possibility of fraud and to test possible theories.

Taylor dismisses radioactive, nuclear or gravitational forces as candidates because none of them could be wielded by a human body with sufficient force to bend a paperclip, let alone a stainless steel spoon. That leaves him with only one of the four natural forces recognized by science – electromagnetism. He pins all his faith on this, suggesting that humans are capable of producing and emitting an 'intentionality field' which interacts with other matter. And he concludes that the phenomena will only be completely understood when we can build a machine to duplicate their effect.

I admire his persistence, but I fear he is destined for disappointment. Any totally materialistic interpretation of reality cannot account for even the best-known properties of the brain such as memory, let alone those effects which have their basis in consciousness. It really is a matter of maintaining balance. We have lost ours by coming down too heavily on the side of technology and reason, and we have begun to pay the price.

But I don't think it is too late to change, too late to listen to our feelings. It seems significant that just at this time, when we most need new answers, all kinds of hints and clues are cropping up everwhere. Some are lost in unlikely places and others are ignored or underestimated simply because they have become distorted by some cult or enthusiasm of which we disapprove. But they are here in abundance right now and, while I would prefer to see us take them seriously, it may not in the end matter how we deal with them. That they exist could be enough.

Just off the coast of Honshu in Japan is a small island called Koshima, where a group of wild macaque monkeys have been under constant observation for more than thirty years. In 1952 their natural diet was supplemented with sweet potatoes spread out on sand at a feeding post. One day in 1953 Imo, an eighteen-month-old female, carried a piece of this food down to a freshwater stream where she washed it, cleaning off the sand under water with her free hand. This made it far more pleasant to eat. She taught the trick to her mother, who showed it to a friendly male and so the habit spread slowly through the colony. At first they used only fresh water but later, again at Imo's instigation, they turned to the sea which not only cleaned the food, but added an interesting new flavour.

This much is clear and well documented in the literature, with researchers watching every step in the spread of the new culture until 1962 when three-quarters of all monkeys over two years old in the Koshima colony were dealing with their food in this way. Then something happened which the resident zoologists perhaps find it hard to come to terms with, for there is great reluctance to talk about it at all.

A point was reached when a certain number of monkeys, let us say ninety-nine, had become enlightened. On two separate islands where colonies were also under observation, similar opportunities had been given to the monkeys, but no such behaviour had ever been seen. Then, one Thursday afternoon at two-fifteen precisely, the hundredth monkey learned the trick. And within half an hour on the other islands, one seventeen and the other twenty-odd miles away, having no direct physical contact with Koshima and no previous history of any such behaviour, all the monkeys suddenly started washing sweet potatoes.

That's the story, and I hope it's true, because it could be the lifeline we need. Looking back at cultural development and the spread of new ideas, it seems that strange things might well work that way. That there is a threshold, a sort of critical mass, for anything new. We talk about an idea 'having its time'. Perhaps this is what we mean. That things grind along until the news reaches the Hundredth Monkey, then in a flash it becomes common knowledge. We see the way towards a new and broader agreement, and the added information or ability passes easily into our heritage.

I hope it is so. I feel at this time, in common with most people in most other disciplines, a great sense of urgency. A sense that time is running out and a suspicion that we are going to have to do something about it for ourselves – and for everything else in the system. We have all the tools we need and all that remains is to find out how best to use them. To make a more sensible agreement about reality. We can do this. Sensibility requires nothing more than attention to all our senses.

To make sense you must have sensed.

That is how it feels to me.

Acknowledgements

The Editor gratefully acknowledges the permission of the following photographers to reproduce their work on the pages listed:

David Beatty   38, 40, 146, 210
Adrian Boot   161
Bill Brandt   53
David Buckland   39
John Bulmer   73 *right*
Lucien Clergue   15
Ira Friedlander   89 (reprinted by permission of Wildwood House)
Mick Gold   152, 160
Ken Heyman   68, 71 *right*, 116, 117, 118
Daniel A. Keintz   45
Richard Lannoy   71 *left*, 248
Norman Loftus   61
C. J. McHugo   158
R. Brian Marsh   145
Roger Mayne   124, 202
David Montgomery   41
Lennart Nilsson   28, 31, 48
Harry Redl   36
Heini Schneebeli   35, 222, 226–229
Harry Shunk   141 (all)
Anthea Sieveking   10, 32, 66–67
Herbert Tichy   90
A. Villani   92.

The photographs on pages 8–9, 16, 22, 25, 26, 34, 37, 44, 54, 58, 60, 108, 111, 177 (both), 180–181, 195–200, 212–216, 218–221 and 256
are by the Editor.

Acknowledgements are also due to:

The Royal Library, Windsor Castle, 78 *bottom* (reproduced by gracious permission of H.M. The Queen); Aerofilms Ltd, 29; the Bettmann Archive Inc., 253 *bottom*; the British Museum, London, 102, 114, 127 (both); *Bunte*, 169; Camera Press, 36, 249; Cleveland Museum of Art, Mr and Mrs William H. Marlatt Fund, 83 (both); Collection Ajit Mookerjee, New Delhi, 236, 237, 241, 242, 246; Collection Jean-Claude Ciancimino, London, 232; Collection John Dugger and David Medalla, London, 239; Collection Mme Nora Martins Lobo, Sofia, 140; Collection Mme René Magritte, Brussels, 73 *left*; Courtauld Institute Galleries, London, 132 *bottom*; Dezo Hoffman Ltd, 156; the Duke of Sutherland Collection, on loan to the National Gallery of Scotland, Edinburgh, 131; Editions Stock, Paris, and Peter Owen Ltd, London, 65; Field Museum of Natural History, Chicago, 135; Professor Richard Gregory, 58–59; Gulbenkian Museum, Durham, 244; Hospital of San Juan Bautista, Toledo, 82 *top*; IBM United Kingdom Ltd, 64; Iveagh Bequest, Kenwood, 133 *left*; Kardorama Ltd, 154; Kasmin, London, 148, 150, 151; Kunsthistorisches Museum, Vienna, 100; the Louvre, Paris, 126, 133 *bottom right*, 182; Mansell-Alinari, 130; Marlborough Fine Art Ltd, London, 47, 115; Mary Evans Picture Library, 253 *top*; Museo Capitolino, Rome, 136–137; Museo de Bellas Artes de Cataluña, Barcelona, 30; Museum of Modern Art, New York, 72, 82 *bottom*, 132 *top* (Lillie P. Bliss Bequest), 144 *bottom*; National Film Archive, London, 97; National Gallery, London, 165; Novosti Press Agency, 251; Philadelphia Museum of Art, the Louise and Walter Arensberg Collection, 147; The Plessey Company Ltd, 29 *bottom*; the Prado, Madrid, 129, 187; Radio Times Hulton Picture Library, 99; Red Dragon Print Collective, 120; Routledge and Kegan Paul Ltd, 81 (from *The Psychology of C. G. Jung*); Schott & Co. Ltd, London, 172, 175; Bani Shorter, 190, 191 (both); Dr Ronald K. Siegel, 42, 43; Stedelijk Museum, Amsterdam, 133 *top right*; *Sunday Times*, London, 41; Uffizi, Florence, 83 *top*; University Books Inc., Secaucus, N.J., 250 *bottom* (from W. Kilner, *The Human Aura*); the Victoria and Albert Museum, London, 33, 123.